MANAGED MENTAL HEALTH SERVICES

MANAGED MENTAL HEALTH SERVICES

By

SAUL FELDMAN, ed.

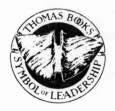

CHARLES C THOMAS • PUBLISHER
Springfield • Illinois • U.S.A.

Published and Distributed Throughout the World by

CHARLES C THOMAS • PUBLISHER
2600 South First Street
Springfield, Illinois 62794-9265

© *1992 by* CHARLES C THOMAS • PUBLISHER

ISBN 0-398-05759-1

Library of Congress Catalog Card Number: 91-834

With THOMAS BOOKS *careful attention is given to all details of manufacturing
and design. It is the Publisher's desire to present books that are satisfactory as to their
physical qualities and artistic possibilities and appropriate for their particular use.*
THOMAS BOOKS *will be true to those laws of quality that assure a good name
and good will.*

Printed in the United States of America
SC-R-3

Library of Congress Cataloging-in-Publication Data

Managed mental health services / by Saul Feldman, ed.
    p.   cm.
    Includes bibliographical references and index.
    ISBN 0-398-05759-1
    1. Mental health services—United States.   2. Managed care plans
(Medical care)—United States.   I. Feldman, Saul.
    [DNLM: 1. Managed Care Programs—organization & administration—
administration—United States.   WM 30 M266]
RA790.6:M29   1991
362.2'0973—dc20
DNLM/DLC
for Library of Congress   91-834
                                                 CIP

To all the Feldmans, present and past,
by birth or affinity, whose esteem and affection
have always been so important to me.

CONTRIBUTORS

Michael J. Bennett, M.D.,
Assistant Clinical Professor of Psychiatry
Harvard Medical School;
Medical Director for Massachusetts
American Biodyne

Jeffrey L. Berlant, M.D., Ph.D.,
Psychiatric Consultant
National Medical Audit,
William Mercer Inc.;
Medical Director
Psychiatric Services,
St. Alphonsus Regional Medical Center

Stephen R. Blum, Ph.D.,
Vice-President
Bay Area Foundation for Human Resources;
Professor of Psychology
California School of Professional Psychology

Richard Frank, Ph.D.,
Professor
School of Hygiene and Public Health
Johns Hopkins University

Gary L. Gaumer, Ph.D.,
Area Manager
Health Research Area
ABT Associates, Inc.

Michael J. Goran, M.D.,
Director
APM, Inc.

Trevor R. Hadley, Ph.D.,
Associate Professor
Department of Psychology
University of Pennsylvania

Richard Kunnes, M.D.,
Chief Operating Officer
U.S. Behavioral Health

Judith R. Lave, Ph.D.,
Professor of Health Economics
University of Pittsburgh

Marvis J. Oehm, M.S.,
Principal
William M. Mercer, Inc.

Joan M. Pearson, Ph.D.,
Consultant
Towers Perrin

J. Peter Rich, Esq.,
Partner
McDermott, Will & Emery

Aileen Rothbard, Sc.D.,
Research Associate
Policy Modeling Workshop
Wharton School
University of Pennsylvania

Arie Schinnar, Ph.D.,
Associate Professor
Policy Modeling Workshop
Wharton School
University of Pennsylvania

Joseph Smith, Ph.D.,
Manager of the Health Policy
Research Program
Workers Compensation Research Institute

H.G. Whittington, M.D.,
Vice President and Medical Director
Managed Health Network, Inc.

Saul Feldman, D.P.A. is Chairman of the Board at U.S. Behavioral Health, a part of The Travelers Corporation. He is also President of the Bay Area Foundation for Human Resources and Editor of the journal, Administration and Policy in Mental Health. Earlier, Dr. Feldman was President of HealthAmerica Corporation of California, Director of the Staff College at the National Institute of Mental Health and Consultant to the World Health and Pan American Health Organizations.

PREFACE

To some observers, *managed* mental health, if not an oxymoron is at least an exercise in futility. The notion that mental health services (particularly those who provide them) are *manageable* defies both logic and experience. Given the complexity of mental health and substance abuse problems, the ideological and conceptual disagreements (someone once said that if asked to form a firing squad, mental health practitioners would get into a circle), the growth in type and number of mental health professionals and the awesome solitude in which they work, the argument is not without merit. In this sense, the term "manage" seems far suited to its archaic meaning "to train a horse in its paces" than to mental health services.

This state of affairs, long true of solo fee-for-service practice, came in the 1980s, to characterize inpatient services as well. The rapid growth of the facilities providing such services has now been well documented. The factors most responsible for this growth include: (1) the relative generosity of inpatient as compared with outpatient mental health and substance abuse benefits, too frequently causing treatment decisions to be unduly influenced by the financial rather than the clinical needs of patients and providers; (2) deregulation and the relaxation of certificate of need requirements that in the past had served as a brake on the expansion of hospitals; (3) the attractive profit margins—almost no dependence by these facilities on public sector reimbursements; (4) declining occupancy rates in general hospitals that caused them to look with uncharacteristic favor on increasing the number of their psychiatric beds; (5) large amounts of investor money seeking opportunities in health care and impressed by the potential returns from psychiatric and substance abuse facilities; and (6) the national attention to substance abuse problems and the well-publicized treatment of celebrities in inpatient facilities.

Not surprising (at least in retrospect), all of this has led to a scenario in which supply stimulates demand, a free market breeds excess rather than efficiency, competition results in higher prices (to retain profit margins, hospital rates have gone up as occupancy rates have gone down), and costs inevitably increase. While there are varied opinions about which of the several cost estimates are correct, the differences are about how much, not whether. By any measure, the increase has been substantial; the only real questions are how much so, whether certain age groups have contributed disproportionately and the like. Given the characteristics of mental health and substance abuse services, the financial incentives to provide the most expensive care in the most intensive places, and the absence of any real accountability, how could it be otherwise?

Whatever the "true" overall cost increases, the major payors for mental health and substance abuse services have come to believe, as a result of their own experience, that costs have been going up much too fast and that something must be done. The point at which the perception of the problem, the "just noticeable difference," converted recognition into concern and concern into action is not clear. Certainly the creation of managed mental health firms eager to develop a market, the advice of health benefits consultants whose work with clients requires them to come up with new ways of doing things, and the formidable publicity about cost increases all played a part.

But the greatest contributors to the development of managed mental health, a development they now bemoan, have been the service providers themselves, practitioners and facilities. By not paying sufficient attention to or not caring about costs and length of treatment, they killed or at least seriously wounded the goose that laid the golden egg, a goose that for them is not likely ever to be as prolific. It is ironic that those who are most unhappy about the advent of managed mental health have done the most to bring it about!

This is not to suggest that the providers of care are necessarily any less virtuous than the managers. The opportunities for excessive self-interest are available to both. The nature of the mental health field—its undefined boundaries, variable technology, uncertain relationship between diagnosis and treatment needs, and unclear success criteria—allows its participants a wide range of discretion, with little proof (or proof easily obtained) of what is "right" and "wrong" behavior.

In such an environment, self-interest and sanctimony are not easily distinguished from altruism and devotion. For care providers and managers alike, the temptation to transform the public's needs into their interests and the patients' problems into their solutions is omnipresent.

For this reason, perhaps more than any other, it is essential that some process be in place that makes more objective, more open and more subject to question, provider decisions about what kind and how much treatment people really need. Such a process, currently called managed care, should, if done properly, help neutralize the power of financial interests (by the provider to do more; by the care manager to do less) and influence clinical decisions. It is this "constructive tension" (a term to which I refer in more detail later) between care provider and manager that probably comes as close as possible to objective decision making in mental health care.

But provider behavior is only one milepost on the road to managed mental health, the one that economists would likely characterize as "supply side." There are others, perhaps less obvious but no less important, others that have at least accelerated the journey. One such is the perceived "success" of managed care in general medicine, at least as a way to contain hospital utilization and costs (though not the overall cost of medical care). The availability of capital and the perception by investors that managed care in mental health represents an interesting "niche" opportunity also played a role. These investors, together with policy-oriented mental health professionals interested in rewards of the "pocket" as well as the "soul," make an unusual but not unprecedented combination: strange bedfellows seeking to do well by doing good.

Stigma and its effect on the use of mental health services is another factor stimulating the growth of managed mental health. Long a barrier to the use of mental health services, stigma appears to be less so than in the past. The "diseasing" of America and its twin, biological psychiatry, i.e., the tendency to attribute substance abuse and mental disorders to biologic, chemical or genetic rather than to personal and environmental factors, has, in my judgment, been a major factor in the decline of stigma, although not intended so.

Whatever its other effects, this ideological voyage toward the "bio" component of the biopsychosocial spectrum of causes and cures appears to be enabling parents and others to escape, at least in part, from the feelings of responsibility and guilt long associated with mental disorders and emotional problems. If a child's disorder is attributable to some organic disease rather than to a dysfunctional home life, for example, then stigma will be less of a barrier and parents will feel more free to seek help for their children.

To borrow a phrase from another field, we appear to have moved into an era of "no-fault" mental disorders. Combined with the lessening of both the time and tolerance of two-career families for coping with the "normal" difficult behavior of adolescents and the attractive appeals of psychiatric and substance abuse hospital advertisements, this "no-fault" mentality appears to be contributing to a decline in stigma and to the overutilization of inpatient services, certainly for children and adolescents. If insurance benefits continue to be far more generous for inpatient than outpatient care and, as a result, hospitalization remains the treatment of financial necessity if not choice for many patients (and financial choice for many providers), this "no-fault" mentality could continue to fuel large increases in inpatient utilization and in costs.

It is, of course, true that the solution to one problem, i.e., the reduction of stigma as a barrier to people getting needed care, almost invariably contains the seeds of another, i.e., people getting too much of the wrong care in the wrong places, a problem that could be even more difficult to resolve than the first. We appear to be experiencing that dilemma and will increasingly so if stigma continues to decline and insurance benefits as well as provider financial incentives remain unchanged. If managed mental health (or something else) does not develop rapidly enough to at least offset these forces, they will, if unchecked, result in continuing high inpatient utilization and we could see cuts in mental health benefits on a scale unprecedented in this country, cuts that could last into the twenty-first century and perhaps beyond.

As managed mental health organizations continue to grow in size and number, their responsibilities and particularly their ethical challenges will grow apace. Not the least of these will be the way they respond to what will inevitably be the increasing competition between them. While I am aware of the arguments in favor of competition (although I have never been entirely persuaded that it is necessarily healthy for health care), more competition could lead to overpromises by some managed mental health firms about how much money they will save potential clients if only they are selected rather than their competitors.

Together with a greater emphasis on profit margins, this overpromise or oversell could begin a cycle difficult to reverse—from overpromise to unrealistically low prices for their services; from low prices to cost cuts for the sake of the "bottom line"; and cost cuts to service cuts. Service cuts could threaten the quality of care; they would most likely be reflected in greater than appropriate restrictions on the use of inpatient care, the area where costs are highest. If this happens, people who truly need such care might not be able to get it. The potential for this kind of pressure and its possible effects must be closely monitored. There is a delicate and difficult to maintain balance between withholding needed care and managing it appropriately.

At its best, managed mental health can improve quality, reduce inappropriate utilization, control costs and protect mental health and substance abuse benefits from a society that has not infrequently been inclined to reduce them. It can also protect individuals, most of whom have benefit limitations, from using up benefits on unnecessary care and then not having any left when care is truly needed.

But at its worst, managed mental health can fall victim to greed, deprive people of services they really need, truncate the role of mental health providers and successfully cut costs but damage the quality of the clinician/patient relationship so central to the success of the therapeutic process.

Managed mental health is now a fact of life and will be increasingly so. It has great potential for doing good, so long as we remain ever mindful of the now immortal words of that greatest of all American philosophers, Charlie Brown, who said "There is no heavier burden than a great potential."

San Francisco, California   Saul Feldman

INTRODUCTION

For managed mental health to flourish, it needs ideas, analyses, research findings and the like—in short, a literature. Much of what has been published so far is probably most accurately (and I hope not too uncharitably) described as strong, if not impassioned opinion—often well expressed but less often well informed. These opinions are helpful; they have contributed to the debate about managed mental health, but too often have generated as much confusion as understanding.

Given the newness of managed mental health, the discomfort it has brought to strong vested interests, and the modest attention it has elicited from academia, the current state of affairs is not surprising. New approaches to mental health services invariably outrun even the most strenuous efforts to understand and improve them; managed mental health is no exception. There is often a considerable lag between action and analysis, implementation and insight. Experienced administrators have learned, and less experienced ones discover (often to their dismay), that in the implementation of new services or new ways of providing old ones, data and research findings are scarce; those that do exist are more useful to justify decisions already made than to help make new ones.

This book is clearly not free of opinion. But we have attempted (readers will judge how successfully) to keep the opinions as informed as possible, based upon the authors' personal experiences in managed mental health and what they know from the experiences of others. Where studies and data do exist, strong efforts have been made to find and incorporate them.

The authors were selected with one major criterion in mind: expertise based on direct experience with managed mental health and the particular subjects about which they have written. Without doubt, their proximity to and identification with managed mental health have skewed them toward the positive. But within this not insignificant constraint, their efforts and those of the editor have been directed toward identifying the problems and negatives as well.

The subjects included are, in the editor's opinion, among the most important to the potential audiences for this book: those involved in or connected to the managed mental health enterprise, i.e., providers, payors, managers, health benefit consultants, human resources and EAP staff; those who have a research/teaching interest in it; and decision makers in the public and private sectors who wonder whether managed mental health is something they should consider.

The choice of subjects in a multi-authored book is never an easy task, limited by a number of factors, not the least of which include the editor's judgment and the availability of knowledgeable authors in a field so new. This latter constraint was, in fact, not much of one at all. The subjects I had in mind and the people willing to write about them matched very well. If readers feel that there are grievous omissions, it is clear where the fault lies.

The chapters range from the genesis of managed mental health, i.e., the general health care context in which it developed (Goran), to its application in particular settings, e.g., the public sector (Hadley), the HMO (Bennett), and the freestanding managed mental health firm (Feldman). The major economic factors fueling its growth are discussed by Frank and Lave and the motivations of managed mental health's most significant purchasers by Kunnes (the insurance carriers) and Pearson (corporate America).

There are few enterprises more information intensive than managed mental health and more dependent on good information systems (Oehm) for efficient operations, for evaluation and for effective quality assurance processes. Smith and Gaumer describe the basic components of a managed mental health evaluation system and the evaluation of the CHAMPUS managed mental health project, the largest to date. Berlant reviews the quality assurance (QA) efforts in general medical care and discusses the special QA needs of the managed mental health organization.

And finally, little new happens in mental health services without raising important clinical, ethical and legal issues. Whittington identifies the clinical rationale for managed mental health, the body of research on which it rests, and its affinity to community mental health. Blum reminds us that managed mental health shares some of the same difficult ethical dilemmas as general health care, but some new and perplexing ones as well. Many of the legal issues (Rich, Martin, and Waldie) are just emerging and are likely to be multi-dimensional: regulatory, malpractice, anti-trust and others. They are adding another component to the already full and complex field of health law.

Absent from the book, and unfortunately so, is a discussion of training. Characteristically, the relationship between new developments in mental health services and the training of those who will implement them is like that of two ships passing in the night—each dimly aware of each other's presence, acknowledging that presence with an occasional blowing of the ship's horn and then passing silently. And after they pass, they continue on their way, unaffected by the brief encounter.

So it is today with managed mental health and the training of mental health professionals. There is little going on; academia has barely taken notice. And yet, managed mental health will depend for its vitality on practitioners and care managers whose training has equipped them to work effectively in this new field.

We need to better understand what is new about managed mental health; how working in it affects clinical practice; what things clinicians should know; how, where and by whom they should be taught and at what point in their careers; and a whole host of other things as well. While clinical training does have a strong generic content, it must help adapt clinical practice to new approaches in providing mental health services. Now we have little to guide us about what these adaptations should be. It does appear that they should include a greater emphasis on such things as short-term goal-oriented psychotherapy, children and adolescents, treatment planning, alternatives to inpatient care, crisis intervention, substance abuse and efficacy, i.e., the relationship between cost and outcome.

But much more than opinion is needed; through studies and analysis we must better understand the interaction between managed mental health and clinical practice and how it should affect the training of mental health professionals. We cannot do so adequately without a dialogue between managed mental health and academia. Otherwise, the performance of managed mental health could have difficulty matching its promise.

Saul Feldman

ACKNOWLEDGMENTS

There is no better vantage point from which to learn and contribute to the development of a new endeavor than that of participant/observer. The founders, funders, owners and staff of U.S. Behavioral Health have made it possible for me and I am grateful to them.

The contributors to this book did so despite heavy responsibilities and many other commitments. I appreciate their willingness to write about so amorphous a field, so early in its life cycle. Without a literature to incite and inform, progress in managed mental health would be much more difficult.

Cindy and Cyd did an outstanding job, deciphering the handwriting of an author/editor who still writes in small letters on large yellow pads.

CONTENTS

MANAGED MENTAL HEALTH SERVICES

Chapter 1

MANAGED MENTAL HEALTH SERVICES: IDEAS AND ISSUES

Saul Feldman

What was until recently a new and perhaps not durable phenomenon with unclear boundaries, undeveloped technology, unexpected visibility and an uncertain future has become a significant factor in the way mental health and substance abuse services are provided in this country. Managed mental health today touches the lives of millions of patients, providers and payors. While there is disagreement about whether it is a malady or a cure, only the most fervent wishful thinking could now consider it as short term or temporary.

With its growing prominence, managed mental health has become a leading topic of discussion in the professional literature and where mental health practitioners gather. Rarely lacking a point of view or the willingness to express it, these practitioners are actively, if not always accurately, contributing to the debate. Managed mental health now appears with regularity on the agendas of meetings all across the country, the major professional organizations have established committees to worry about it, and their publications are replete with impassioned letters to the editor as well as more objective articles. If not yet the most visible or controversial issue affecting mental health services, it may soon be.

Like other changes with significant economic consequences, managed mental health seems to be generating more heat than light, more rhetoric than reason. It is coming to be seen as a solution, if not a panacea, by its advocates and as a menace by its adversaries, particularly the private for-profit psychiatric and substance abuse hospital chains whose fortunes blossomed in the 1980s and who are understandably upset by anything that could hurt their revenues. Their unhappiness is not based simply on anxiety about the future. Managed mental health has already damaged not only their prospects but their current financial well being.

Attendees at the 1991 annual meeting of the National Association of

Private Psychiatric Hospitals, heard a speaker suggest that "The current and growing crisis in hospital psychiatry is felt by many to be a struggle for survival" (Lewis, 1991). In February 1991, Charter Medical Corporation, the largest owner of private for-profit psychiatric hospitals in America, in a letter to the "employee health benefits community" wrote "The dramatic and fundamental changes in the mental health care industry have had a negative impact on business." The letter goes on to indicate that Charter would attempt to adapt to the changes in the mental health field by making "Charter the provider of choice among managed care firms and insurance companies."

Referring to inpatient substance abuse facilities, *The Wall Street Journal* concluded that "Substance abuse treatment is no longer a growth industry. After years of brisk expansion ... (they) are struggling to cope with falling occupancy rates and pressures to lower their charges" (Bacon, 1990). And *Healthweek* reported that "Woes mount for addiction services firms as Parkside Med shuts down half of its centers" (Kirshner, 1990). Such reports have become almost commonplace in the public and professional media.

But the inpatient programs are not the only unhappy ones. Even the most casual glance through the newsletters and other publications of the major professional associations (particularly the psychiatrists) suggests the intensity of their feelings. The headline of an article in the January 1990 issue of *Psychiatric News,* for example, stated that "Trustees attack managed care threat." The April 1990 issue of the *American Psychologist* refers to the "Mental Health Care Revolution" and asks "Will Psychologists Survive?" (Zimet, 1990). These and other publications are replete with advice to their members about how to cope with the threat (and more subtly) with the opportunity presented by managed mental health.

Not surprisingly, the articles and reports from the business community have a different tone. *The Wall Street Journal,* for example, reported that " ... a subsidiary of the Halliburton Company saw its costs for mental health and substance abuse treatment drop $590,000 in this year's first quarter after it adopted a managed care plan" (Bacon, 1990). A number of major insurance carriers and other companies have reported large savings as a result of managed mental health programs, as high as 50% (England, 1989).

These reports and many others like them suggest that managed mental health is having an effect on the cost of mental health and substance abuse services. The extent to which these hopeful data (perhaps combined with the desire to avoid more painful alternatives) have influenced the behavior of self-insured employers and insurance carriers all across the country, is illustrated by the rapid growth of managed mental health programs.

Money and Power

There is little doubt that the rush toward managed care in mental health has been inspired by the well documented and fearsome increases in the cost of mental health and substance abuse services during the past decade. But the debate about managed mental health is not entirely about money, although its economic effects are important. It is also about professional prerogatives, about power and about autonomy, things that most mental health professionals value so highly but do not often admit. Both the economic and power concerns are real—as managed mental health continues to grow, it will bring about major changes in the financial status quo and in the way hospitals and practitioners go about doing their business.

Since money and power appear to evoke greater passion than ideology, the rhetoric about managed mental health may well get more heated before long. At the same time, money and power are not things that are ordinarily discussed or argued about openly, at least not by mental health professionals. They tend to deny or at least not acknowledge their self-interest while actively pursuing it and give the impression that they view money and power very "much like the Victorian view of sex. It is seen as vulgar, as a sign of character defect, as something an upstanding professional would not be interested in or stoop to engage in" (Levinson and Klerman, 1972).

So the dialogue about managed mental health is often framed in terms that are more professionally and socially acceptable—terms such as "quality of care," "professional standards" and "patient needs." And certainly, any time a change of any consequence to patient care takes place, its effects on quality must be addressed and closely examined. But not surprisingly, those whose financial and power needs are threatened seem somehow to see change as bad for the quality of care and the status quo as good, or at least better (*Psychiatric News*, 1989). And financial interests are at stake here. The emphasis in managed mental health so far is on people who are employed and who have mental health benefits, a population very attractive to mental health providers.[1] Managed mental health programs already control access to services for millions of such people throughout the country and the number is growing rapidly.

For some, perhaps many mental health professionals, the change in the power relationships brought about by managed care is at least as distressing as the economics. It chips away at what many of them hold most dear and most zealously try to protect: their professional autonomy. The ability (or divine right) to be free of all controls over their behavior is highly cherished by mental health professionals, particularly but certainly not exclusively by physicians. I have used the term "M. Deity" as a perhaps uncharitable description of this attitude in physicians. "Ph. Deity" is closely related (Feldman, 1978).

These two dimensions, i.e., its effect on the financial well-being of providers and its "intrusion" into clinical decisions that have historically been the almost exclusive domain of patients and practitioners, primarily the latter, have engendered the most opposition to managed mental health, the most concern and the most heated opinions.

Justified Criticism

Because managed mental health has not been around very long, there has been little in the way of dispassionate analysis and research. By and large, the professional literature is still a collection of anecdotes and observations that tend to reflect the optimism of those who are doing managed mental health and the unhappiness of those it is being done to: practitioners and hospitals whose lives are changing for the worse, at least from their perspective.

But it would be a mistake to conclude that the animosity toward managed mental health is simply a reflection of bruised egos and economic self-interest. Some of the negativism about it is well justified by the behavior of some managed mental health firms. Managed mental health is not a uniform, fixed process—it comes in a number of different shapes and sizes and it is these differences that determine its quality. There are utilization managers, for example, who are not sufficiently well trained or competent to do their jobs adequately. They appear incapable of much more than a rote recitation from protocols of dubious

---

1. The public sector is beginning to awaken to the potential of managed care as a way to make mental health services under Medicaid more cost-effective. This may well emerge as a major shift in the way such services are provided in the future.

value about whether the condition of a particular patient warrants an inpatient admission. These extremely important judgments about the locus and type of care to be provided to patients are often made by telephone over long distances. Even for well trained clinician/utilization managers, informed responsible decisions are not easily made. For those less trained, it may not be possible, particularly if there is a strong bias against inpatient care.

Some (hopefully not many) managed mental health firms do appear to have an overly strong bias (ideological and financial) against inpatient care, and try too hard to find reasons for denying inpatient admissions and reducing lengths of stay. In such cases, they may use their power injudiciously, at the expense of good patient care. Where mental health providers have come into contact with such practices, their criticisms are justified, but too often generalized to the entire managed mental health field.

Too frequently, managed mental health is essentially the equivalent of utilization review in which provider claims for payment are reviewed to determine whether hospital admissions and lengths of stay are/were appropriate. This type of review, a carryover from general medical care, depends heavily on fixed protocols and norms and is generally done by telephone.

But even in the hands of qualified reviewers, norms and protocols are simply no substitute for clinical judgments based upon familiarity with the patients' needs and social situation as well as with the available treatment alternatives. While managed mental health, by its very nature, intrudes into the decision making process between patient and clinician, the quality of the intrusion must be such as to justify its existence.

Done properly, managed mental health should essentially be a system of checks and balances, including such activities as pre-treatment authorization, concurrent and retrospective utilization review, care management, claims review and quality assurance. Clinical and administrative expertise are combined with financial incentives to providers and consumers to help make mental health services more cost-effective.

Managed mental health should be a method to better match the treatment to the problem, recognizing the uncertain relationship between diagnosis and treatment as well as the subjective nature of clinical decisions in mental health. Good managed mental health programs should integrate managers, providers and payors into a system of care that reflects an understanding of the special needs and characteristics of the mental health field.

Perhaps the loudest and most impassioned criticisms of managed mental health have centered on quality, that managed mental health is lowering and perhaps seriously damaging the quality of care provided to those in a managed system. As used in this context, quality tends to be equated with quantity and locus, i.e., patients are getting too little care or at least less than they need and are too frequently getting it outside of rather than in the hospital.

Given the methodological problems inherent in mental health services research, it is far too early to demonstrate with any degree of accuracy the extent to which these criticisms are valid. But they all tend to at least imply that patients (and presumably providers although this is much less emphasized) are being victimized by a system in which there are few if any protections for them and constraints against the behavior of the care managers. These criticisms are not unfamiliar; they closely resemble those that were leveled with equal passion against HMOs in earlier days. They are also untrue.

Safeguards

What the critics seem to overlook or at least not acknowledge are the safeguards against abuse in a managed mental health system, safeguards that protect patients and assure quality far beyond what is possible in unmanaged care. Many employers, for example, closely monitor the activities of the managed mental health firms they have selected. The processes they use to do so include confidential employee satisfaction surveys and an analysis of complaints they receive from employees and dependents dissatisfied with their care. Employees are encouraged to report such concerns promptly. These and other issues are discussed regularly with the managed care firm. And most firms have highly visible complaint systems. Complaints are taken seriously, investigated and reported to the employer, many of whom require it. To whom do patients in an unmanaged system complain? And with what effect? How much leverage do they have?

Some employers use outside experts to review and evaluate the care provided. Pacific Telesis, for example, has used a national medical audit group for that purpose. A team of experienced mental health professionals does a comprehensive on site audit that includes a review of records, quality standards, staff qualifications, and the care management process. IBM uses a panel of outside mental health experts to review, on an ongoing basis, the work done by its managed mental health firm. (A whole new growth area may be opening up for mental health professionals—consultants to employers to monitor the work of managed mental health firms who in turn monitor the work of mental health professionals.)

Providers have not been reluctant to report to employers and directly to the managed mental health firms what they consider to be inappropriate practices. These complaints are taken seriously and are investigated. Managed mental health firms also have an appeals process for providers who are unhappy about the decisions of utilization managers. While the processes vary, they generally include a final decision by the medical director if the issue is not resolved at a lower level. When they occur, disagreements are most often about locus of care, i.e., whether the care should be in or out of the hospital. The professional associations actively encourage complaints about managed care from their members. In its biweekly publication, the American Psychiatric Association, for example, has a very prominent regular announcement on the front page soliciting complaints about managed mental health from psychiatrists.

Many employers, particularly large ones, decide to use a managed mental health firm on the advice of an outside consulting group. These consultants also play a significant role in the process through which a particular firm is selected. They often use staff or outside mental health professionals to help them. Their future business prospects are very much affected by their ability to help select the "right" managed mental health firm and to help make certain the one they select does a good job. It is also clearly in the best interest of the managed mental health firm to do so, if it wants to be recommended by the consulting group to other prospective clients.

The values, standards and professionalism of the clinician/care managers employed by the managed mental health firm and the practitioners with whom they interact have the most profound effect on the quality of the services provided under managed mental health. The practitioners who actually provide the direct services (excluding at least for the moment those who are employed directly by the staff model managed mental health firms) are not at all reticent to express their points of view about the care of patients for whom they are responsible. They do not passively accept the judgment of the managed care firm (nor should they) when it conflicts with their own about what is best for the patient. After all, they are the ones who have the most direct contact with patients. They have a significant effect on the clinical decisions that are ultimately made.

The care managers or reviewers employed by the managed mental health firms are themselves (or should be) well-trained mental health professionals who, while inevitably influenced by the contexts in which they work, are unlikely to be coopted by them. They have strong allegiances to the values and ethics of their professions. It has long been true that professionals tend to be more identified with and loyal to the standards of their professions and the associations to which they belong than to the organizations by which they are employed (Raelin, 1986). These allegiances and the professionalism of the care managers help neutralize any undue influence on their behavior by the managed mental health firm.

Constructive Tension

The interaction or constructive tension between the two—practitioner and clinician/care manager—should have an important and positive effect on the quality of care in the managed system. But this is not always the case. Constructive tension between the two is only possible where the direct patient care is provided by practitioners who are not overly dependent on the managed mental health firm for referrals and therefore, for their economic well being. In this sense it is essential for managed mental health firms to have a sufficiently large network of practitioners so that the dependency relationships are in proper balance. It is not clear whether there is a "magic number" but as a general guideline, it is probably best that no single managed mental health firm be responsible for more than 15–20% of any individual clinician's practice.

If the constructive tension is to work in the best interests of the patient, the independence of the practitioners who provide the direct services must be maintained. Where the managed mental health firm controls too much of an individual clinician's practice or where it employs clinicians directly (the staff model), the dependency relationship is such that clinicians may be (often not consciously) overly inclined to please and to comply with what they perceive to be the firm's implied or explicit wishes. There is some question, therefore, about whether it is wise for managed mental health firms to employ their own clinical staff as the direct service providers. While they gain control and perhaps efficiency, they may lose the constructive tension, the checks and balances that are so important to quality. Such control exacerbates the potential conflict of interest in being both the manager and provider of care.

These safeguards do not guarantee that mental health care under a managed system will be free of bad practice, and it is not. But nothing as impressive in magnitude or kind exists in unmanaged mental health, where laissez faire prevails and protections against bad practice, where they exist at all, do so only at the extremes. In managed mental health, the safeguards against improper practice are far more extensive, better developed and therefore much more likely to insulate the care of patients from the self serving behavior of providers and managers.

Benefit Flexibility and Protection

But safeguarding quality and reducing unnecessary expenditures, while perhaps the most obvious are not the only positive effects of managed mental health. It has encouraged payors—insurance carriers and self-insured employers—to provide much more benefit flexibility than has ever before been the case. The mental health and substance abuse benefits provided by payors under managed care are significantly more flexible and there is far greater benefit substitution than in unmanaged programs.

The lack of benefit flexibility (the range and scope of benefits provided as well as the ability to substitute one for another) has long been a perplexing problem in the mental health field. It has been a major reason for the very slow growth of alternatives to inpatient care in the United States. While inpatient psychiatric coverage is available to over 90% of employees with health benefits, coverage for alternatives to inpatient care is difficult to find. While these programs have long been acknowledged as effective and much less expensive than 24-hour inpatient care for many patients, payors have been concerned that they would not be used as substitutes for inpatient care but rather as additions to and, therefore, if they were covered, costs would go up even more. This rationale is, of course, in addition to the traditional reluctance of payors to expand benefits for mental health at all. Managed care has brought with it major changes in mental health benefits and greater benefit flexibility as payors discover that in a well managed system, these benefits are truly cost effective substitutes for much more expensive hospitalization.

Another important by product of managed mental health is benefit protection. It is almost always the case that mental health and substance abuse benefits are far more limited than are those for general medical care. These limits are often stated in maximum dollar amounts allowable annually and/or over a lifetime. If the limited benefits are used up on expensive and unnecessary inpatient care, and as is not infrequently the case, further treatment is required at a later time, there may be little or no benefit left to pay for it. The alternatives then are to forego needed care, pay for it out of pocket or seek it in the public sector. Since the alternatives to inpatient care generally cost only about 35% of a typical inpatient stay, a lot more of the benefit remains; if care is needed again, it is available.

A CASE EXAMPLE

U.S. Behavioral Health (USBH) is one of the better known managed mental health organizations in the country. While not a prototype, its development and operations may help illustrate at least one approach to the field. Founded in the late 1970s as an employee assistance company, it began to develop a comprehensive managed mental health and substance abuse program in 1988 with funding from private investors.

What the investors saw and what interested them in managed mental health were rapidly growing costs and inpatient utilization, thriving private psychiatric and substance abuse inpatient facilities, and clinicians in private practice working in splendid isolation, with little regard for costs and efficacy. What they also saw were the substantial inroads of managed care in general medicine and its inevitable application to mental health.

What came to pass at USBH was a combination of investors seeking capital growth, policy-oriented mental health professionals, many with community mental health backgrounds, and others interested in creating and profiting from an organized care system to help prevent the erosion of mental health and substance abuse benefits that would inevitably result from excessive inpatient utilization and costs. This combination of interests at USBH was not atypical—the motivations and agendas that led to its creation were not dissimilar from those of other managed mental health organizations.

Basic Assumptions

The programs we developed at USBH rest on some basic assumptions and beliefs about managed care and the mental health field in general. We believe that the keys to quality, cost-effective mental health services are easy accessibility, early intervention, a comprehensive care management system that ensures continuity, and high quality, cost-conscious providers who believe that it is better to treat patients in the community than in the hospital whenever appropriate and who value short term goal-oriented psychotherapy.

We believe that mental health and substance abuse problems are contagious—that they inevitably affect other family members—and that they are generally not self-limiting as are so many medical problems. Rather, they get worse if unattended, requiring more intensive care at much greater cost later on and cause high use of expensive medical services. We believe that too many people get inpatient care who do not need it; are using up their limited benefits on unnecessary care; and are being removed from work and family to get that care. We believe that through collaboration between providers, patients, payors and care managers, good care at a reasonable cost is achievable and mental health benefits can be protected.

We believe that mental health and substance abuse services are better for people when providers of care work in a system where accountability enhances rather than detracts from the virtues of autonomy; that clinicians with too little autonomy threaten good patient care no less than those with too much; and that the best outcomes for patients come from checks and balances, from a blend of expertise and motivations.

Care Management Process

As do other managed mental health organizations, USBH works with self-insured employers, insurance carriers, union trusts, HMOs and others to manage the mental health and substance abuse benefits to which their employees or members are entitled. Those within our managed care system seek help by calling us on 24-hour toll free lines. Their calls are taken by masters level clinical staff employed by USBH whose job it is to understand the presenting problems and to engage the callers in such a way as to help them accept a first appointment, wherever possible. The goal is to enhance access. It reflects our conviction that if identified early, problems can be dealt with much more effectively and at a much lower cost, both financially and with regard to human suffering. We also recognize how fragile and tentative that first call for help often is.

We learn enough about the caller's situation to make a referral for an in-person assessment and where appropriate, for brief outpatient psychotherapy with one of our network practitioners. Because we have a computerized profile on every practitioner in our network, we are able to match the callers' problems and demographic characteristics with the location and particular expertise of our practitioners to make the most appropriate referral. Practitioners are expected to offer an appointment to take place within 72 hours of the time they are called, except in urgent situations.

The assessments and brief (usually less than 10 sessions) psychotherapy are done in their own offices by practitioners under contract to USBH. They are experienced clinicians, skilled in diagnosis, treatment planning and treatment. They are in solo or small group practices and become part of our provider network following a review of their qualifications. They must agree to work within a structure that emphasizes collaboration, accountability and joint decision making as well as an ongoing review of the quality of their work. USBH has a credentials committee composed of outside mental health professionals who help us develop the standards we use to select network providers and to review the applications from those who desire to join.[2]

If in the clinician's judgment more than 10 treatment sessions will be required, a call is made to one of the USBH care managers and jointly the clinician and care manager make a decision about the need for further treatment. The care managers are licensed, experienced mental health professionals—psychologists, psychiatric social workers and psychiatric nurses. They are employed by USBH and backed up by clinical supervisors and two full-time psychiatrists, one of whom is the medical director and the other a specialist in child and adolescent mental health.

The care managers have at least 10 years of clinical experience in

---

2. We are aware that even the best conceived and implemented selection processes and standards do not guarantee that all practitioners selected will be well enough qualified. Good practitioner networks evolve—a careful selection must be followed by an ongoing and rigorous evaluation process in which practitioners are rated on such criteria as responsiveness to patient needs, the quality of their assessments and treatment plans, the efficacy of their interventions and the like. In most areas of the country, the number of practitioners applying to join our network is greater than our need. There has been a large increase in such applicants during the past three years, an acknowledgement by practitioners, in some cases begrudging, that managed mental health is growing and may be around for awhile.

residential and outpatient settings as well as in substance abuse and mental health. Because of this experience (for many including private practice as well) they are able to interact as peers with the providers in our network. The interaction is not unlike a collegial discussion between two competent professionals discussing a patient. While the clinical skills and experience of the discussants are similar, their orientations are generally different, i.e., the network practitioners are likely to have a fee-for-service, more is better perspective while the USBH care managers will generally feel that less (intensive and expensive) is better. Out of this constructive tension, this interaction between competent clinicians with often different perspectives and financial inclinations comes clinical decisions that are probably as close to truth and objectivity as is possible in the mental health field.

USBH also contracts with licensed psychiatric hospitals and substance abuse facilities, structured outpatient programs and other alternatives to inpatient care where they exist.[3] They must agree to cooperate with our care management system. These facilities are site visited by our clinical staff to make certain that they are of sufficiently high quality.

Quality and Cost Saving

The care managers are responsible for tracking and reviewing the treatment being provided. They are in ongoing contact with practitioners and facilities to be certain that patients are not falling through the cracks, that they are getting the care they need, that sufficient progress is being made, and that resources are being used appropriately. When inpatient treatment is needed, the care managers authorize it (in concert with one of our psychiatrists) and collaborate in developing the treatment and discharge plan. They are also responsible for arranging aftercare (all patients in substance abuse treatment are referred to an aftercare program after their formal treatment and are followed up for a year).

Quality assurance activities include the credentialing process used in provider selection, ongoing and intensive supervision of in-house clinical staff, case conferences, focused and random audits, patient satisfaction surveys and an active program of staff and network practitioner

---

3. While it is less true now than in the past, it is still difficult to find an adequate number of community alternatives to inpatient care—day care, partial hospitalization and the like. As managed mental health grows, however, the number of such programs will grow apace since managed care brings with it the flexibility, benefit substition and therefore, the money that makes such growth possible.

education. The quality assurance activities are supervised by our psychiatrist medical director and by a quality assurance committee composed of our own staff and a majority of outside practitioners. We also have a Board of Scientific Advisors composed of members prominent in mental health and substance abuse, and in a particular area of specialization, e.g., child mental health, psychopharmacology, long term care, evaluation research, training, to be certain that our services and policies continue to reflect the most current thinking in the field.

Our experience shows that compared with unmanaged care, substantial cost savings, often as high as 40% or more can be achieved. The major savings result from negotiated rates with practitioners (about 20% less than their customary charges) and with facilities, but primarily from reduced inpatient utilization, not from reductions in outpatient care. In many cases, outpatient care is increased beyond what would ordinarily be provided in an unmanaged system. According to Broskowski (1990) "It is not uncommon to observe an increase in the number of outpatient users and . . . in the average number of outpatient visits per episode at the same time that unnecessary inpatient care is reduced." Given the high inpatient utilization in unmanaged care (about 120 days per thousand persons per year and in many companies much higher) impressive savings are clearly possible. For outpatient care, the emphasis is on short-term approaches. We are not likely to authorize psychoanalysis or long-term psychoanalytic psychotherapy unless it can be demonstrated as "medically necessary" (Michels, 1990). The goal is functional improvement and symptom reduction, not personality reconstruction.

Most of what we do at U.S. Behavioral Health rests on existing research findings that for the great majority of patients, alternatives to inpatient care are at least as effective and far less expensive. Managed mental health is, in effect, a new application of research findings and clinical approaches that have been around for some time. Its basic concepts and technology rest on a large and well documented body of research and practice as well as an ideology (particularly congenial to community mental health), none of which are really new. Simply put, it suggests that all but a relatively few people with mental and substance abuse disorders can be treated and maintained outside of the hospital, at least as effectively and at a much lower cost. When hospitalization is necessary, it should be as brief as possible. Even detoxification, long considered as absolutely requiring hospitalization, is no longer for many patients (Hayoshida et. al., 1989).

What is new about managed mental health is the extent to which it has found acceptance in the market place as a solution to a difficult set of problems, the organizations by which it is provided, and its ability to incorporate financial incentives against overutilization. For the first time in any significant way, at least in the mental health field, the ideology of community care and the financial imperative to provide it have coalesced. The traditional and pervasive financial incentives to provide the most expensive care in the most intensive places are beginning to erode as managed mental health takes hold.

Examples are not difficult to find. One of our clients at USBH, a large self insured company with more than 50,000 employees, implemented a new substance abuse benefit as an outcome of collective bargaining. In the first year of the program, about 70% of the employees and dependents who used the benefit got care in a 28-day inpatient program at an average cost of about $10,000 per stay. The company was concerned about the costs, about whether so much inpatient care was really necessary or desirable and about its ability to continue to fund the program. Its benefit consultants, a large well respected firm, suggested managed care as a way to contain the costs and help ensure that the care would be provided in the most appropriate places. USBH was awarded the contract and paid a management fee for its services.[4]

In the first year under the contract, the utilization pattern was reversed; 70% of those who used the benefit in that year (and in subsequent years as well) were treated in a structured outpatient program and then in community aftercare programs. The company saved a lot of money, the benefit was retained and the recidivism rate (as measured by "clean and sober" for one year following treatment) dropped. The utilization and cost reductions achieved in the first year of the contract have been maintained in subsequent years.

What caused these changes (not at all atypical), was not the discovery of some new treatment or diagnostic procedures but simply the motivation and skill to apply what was already well known and well documented; to do a good clinical job; to provide care in the community wherever possible; and in the process to protect employee benefits and save money.

---

4. Managed mental health firms are generally paid in two ways: A fee for their services or a "risk" arrangement similar to that of an HMO in which what they earn depends upon the difference between what they are paid and the cost of the services provided. Newer forms of payment, often a blend of these two basic approaches, are also used.

The amount of waste and unnecessary care in the previously unmanaged program were so flagrant that even if saving money had not been one of the motivations, it would have taken place anyway.

FUTURE CHALLENGES

But what about the future? While there is little reason to doubt the wisdom of the old Chinese proverb that says "To worry about tomorrow is to be unhappy today" some speculation about the future can, on occasion, at least stimulate if not inform debate.

Need For Research

The number of people whose mental health care is managed has been growing rapidly. It is not yet possible to estimate with any accuracy what the number actually is. There is not so far a systematic effort in place to collect such data, and even if there were, its success might be limited. By and large, the large managed mental health programs are operated by private for-profit firms. In a competitive environment, they are not likely to be enthusiastic about providing data that could help illuminate the extent, nature and perhaps effects of their services. While competition in health care may have other virtues, data sharing, information exchange and the like, to an extent that would enhance research, are generally not among them.

But there is little doubt that the growth has been rapid and broad—by geography, industry, client type and size. It appears that large employers are more involved in managed mental health than are smaller ones. They generally have more comprehensive benefits, significant unions involvement (health benefits are increasingly a collective bargaining issue) and they use consultants who evaluate and frequently advocate the adoption of a managed mental health program. At least in part due to more generous benefits, their mental health and substance abuse costs have been higher (Higgins, 1990).

Not surprisingly, the rapid growth of managed mental health has left in its wake a number of important, unattended and unresolved issues. As the field matures, a literature will develop and at least some of the issues will be addressed, if not resolved. Before much more time goes by, the practices and policies of managed mental health must be informed by research and by reasonably dispassionate analyses. To do so, will require a willingness on the part of the managed mental health firms to share statistical and experiential data. With appropriate safeguards built in to protect the confidentiality of proprietary information, such research should be possible and must be done.

Effect on Benefits

A major issue will continue to be the one that caused the emergence of managed mental health in the first place: the utilization of services and its effect on costs and benefits. As discussed earlier, where managed mental health programs have been implemented, their effects on in-patient utilization and on costs are visible and impressive. Ordinarily, this cost containment would accelerate or at least continue as managed mental health grows and covers more people.

But there are other forces at work, ones that could well change this scenario. Some inpatient facilities appear, perhaps temporarily, to be reacting to falling occupancy rates by raising prices, by heavier than usual promotions to increase patient referrals, by the use of such things as *under-utilization* review committees, by incentives to staff and to clinicians to increase admissions and to prolong lengths of stay, by extending admitting privileges to nonmedical mental health professionals and the like. In short, they appear to be doing many of the same things, only more of them, that caused the growth of managed mental health in the first place.

If these efforts succeed, they could offset, at least partially, the cost containment effects beginning to be achieved by managed mental health programs still in their infancy, and costs could continue their upward spiral at least until (and inevitably) benefits are cut as a last resort. And benefit cuts are already taking place. According to the Bureau of Labor Statistics, "77% of the nation's employers in 1989 were imposing more restrictive conditions on hospitalization for mental illness and chemical dependency than other medical insurance benefits; in 1980, 44% were doing so" (*Los Angeles Times*, 1991). During the same period, cuts in outpatient benefits were deep and widespread.

Other hospitals appear to be reacting more positively: developing new programs as alternatives to inpatient care, more responsible promotion efforts, and fixed cost financial arrangements that do not reward unnecessarily long lengths of stay. These are obviously the facilities with which managed mental health firms are most likely to work.

It is not yet clear which of these behaviors will prevail. One way or the other, it seems inevitable that the cost increases of the past will moderate and decline through the efforts of managed mental health, changes in provider behavior or most unfortunately, benefit cuts.

Alternatives to Inpatient Care

In this decade, there is likely to be a more rapid development of alternatives to inpatient care than has ever been true before. The growth of managed mental health if it continues, will bring about a new environment, one in which benefits are revised and money becomes available to pay for such programs, as has never been true in the past. Managed mental health and alternative programs to inpatient care are natural partners. It is unfortunately the case that too few such programs are available now and too often hospitalization becomes necessary for patients who could otherwise avoid it. As a result, even patients within managed care programs are being hospitalized unnecessarily because of the unavailability of alternatives and costs are higher than would otherwise be the case.

Quality

The growth of managed mental health has brought with it a heightened discussion about issues of quality. To some extent, this interest derives from the rhetoric of those who are unhappy about managed mental health: clinicians and facilities who criticize it as eroding the quality of care because it is "depriving" people of care they truly need in the interest of saving money. The advocates of managed mental health take the opposite point of view and the debate, almost entirely uninformed by research, goes on.

There is at this juncture little evidence for the critics or advocates to use in their arguments about whether managed mental health is good or bad for the quality of care. But the intensity of the debate is likely to spark a great deal more attention to issues of quality, in part because of the size to which managed mental health will grow, in part because of the accusations from its adversaries, and in part because of the legitimate interest of clients, providers, managers of care and payors. Quality and efficacy will become more important issues than in the past.

Attempts to assess and ensure quality are likely to take two major forms: increasing calls for regulation of managed care and demands for studies, data and the like to serve as the basis for assessing quality. The regulation approach is clearly picking up steam. Stimulated in no small part by general acute care hospitals unhappy with utilization review, state legislatures are turning to regulation and by 1990, approximately 11 states had enacted such legislation (Open Minds, 1990). The trend seems likely to continue although it is unlikely, at least in mental health, to have much of an effect on quality, aside from its most egregious and obvious aspects.

State regulation is also making it more likely that utilization management firms will make public the criteria by which they make decisions about inpatient admissions and lengths of stay. There has grown up in the medical field (and increasingly so in mental health) the notion that somehow the criteria and protocols used in utilization management are the critical elements in decisions about locus and length of care and have an important effect on quality. This belief has developed, at least in part, out of the promotional efforts of some managed mental health firms who in their marketing efforts glorified the importance and uniqueness of their protocols as the "block box" solution to the overutilization problem.

Much more important than the criteria—often quite general and of limited value, particularly in mental health—are the people and processes through which treatment decisions are made. Criteria are much more effectively used as guides to rather than determinants of such decisions. Those who most fervently advocate the publication of such protocols are likely to discover before too long that like the Wizard of Oz, they are much less formidable than they appear.

The growth of managed mental health is beginning to highlight outcome, one particular aspect of quality that has probably been too little emphasized in the past, i.e., the extent to which services have resulted in some functional improvement, both at home and at work for people receiving care and whether the improvement was worth the cost. This emphasis on quality as the improvement of function is closely related to efficacy, an attempt to better understand the relationship between cost and outcome in an attempt to address such questions as what was accomplished with the resources used? Was it "worth it" and how can we tell? Questions of this type have been conspicuous by their absence from mental health and health care (Relman, 1988).

Provider Attitudes

In the final analysis, the quality of mental health and substance abuse services will be determined as it always has been, by the behavior of providers—clinicians and facilities. It is in the consulting rooms, the treatment centers and the hospitals where such things are truly decided. The effects of managed mental health on that behavior may well be one of the most important quality issues in the 1990s. The challenge is to help providers better understand and identify with the concepts and goals of managed mental health, not simply to reward and punish through financial incentives.

If too many providers become and stay involved in managed mental health simply for economic reasons or because they are afraid not to, and assume that they will continue to practice as if nothing has changed, quality will be undermined. There is little doubt that most providers who sign on initially with managed mental health do so to expand or at least protect their referrals. But if managed mental health works as it should and demonstrates its contribution to cost containment, benefit protection and quality, providers will come to identify with it for more than financial reasons. This issue, the extent to which increasing numbers of providers will subscribe to the ideology and goals of managed mental health will be a significant one in the 1990s.

There is reason for optimism, given the experience of HMOs. Early in their development, it was difficult for many of them to convince practitioners and hospitals to sign contracts and provide care for their patients. But in just a few years, the relationship shifted and hospitals as well as physicians were eager to do so. While their interest was initially and for some time thereafter primarily economic, that began to change and is still in the process of doing so.

This is not to suggest that the antipathy by providers for HMOs has disappeared or that economics does not still play a significant role in their motivation to work with HMOs. It is fair to say, however, that experience with HMOs, research studies about the quality of care in HMOs as compared with fee-for-service medicine, and other factors have caused many practitioners to look more benignly at the HMO not only as a provider and manager of care but as an employer as well. It is not unlikely that the same process will take place (and appears to already be doing so) in managed mental health. Managed mental health firms are experiencing a dramatic improvement in their ability to contract with experienced, qualified providers throughout the country, in all the mental health disciplines.

Checks and Balances

I referred earlier to "checks and balances," i.e., the constructive tension between the care manager and practitioner when they interact around such issues as treatment planning and the locus of care. This interaction between well qualified professionals with somewhat different perspectives can lead, in my judgment, to the best clinical decisions. But checks and balances only work well when the parties to the process are independent, neither being overly dominant. There may be a danger to this somewhat precarious balance if as managed mental health grows, practitioners become too dependent on them for referrals and therefore too likely to please and defer to them. In such an event, the constructive tension that I believe is so healthy may lessen or disappear, to the detriment of the patient's care and the practitioner's autonomy.

Constructive tension requires self discipline on the part of practitioners and care managers. For practitioners, it means resisting the temptation through overly compliant behavior, to gain a favored position with the managed mental health firm vis-à-vis referrals. As the number of practitioners and therefore the competition for patients continues to grow, and managed mental health comes to control access to mental health and substance abuse services for a larger and larger number of people, the temptation to please will become more compelling.

For the manager of care, the temptation to resist will be excessive control over practitioner behavior; the efficiency, ease of operations and enhanced profitability (at least in the short term) that may come from working with dependent, compliant practitioners. If the seduction (of both parties) takes place, it will be at the expense of good patient care. Managed mental health firms need to be alert to this possibility and to guard against it. It will be an important responsibility of their growing power.

The extent to which the proper dependency balance between care manager and practitioner can be maintained depends, at least in part, on the way the managed mental health firm is structured. Some refer patients whose care they manage to independent clinicians in private practice or in organized care settings. For these practitioners, patient referrals from the managed mental health firm constitute only one source of their revenue. How significant a source that should be, and at what point if any it alters the dependency relationship in a way that could be inimical to good patient care is not clear.

What is clear, however, is the need to preserve the freedom of these practitioners to disagree, to question and to ultimately disengage themselves from managed mental health programs that they truly believe are not working in the best interest of patients. The point at which this freedom is threatened will of course vary between practitioners but it is an issue to which managed mental health firms must be sensitive. This is not to suggest that such relationships should be stressful but rather to emphasize the importance of independent practitioners—challenging, questioning and disagreeing in the interest of good patient care. Care managers must understand and remember how easy it is to mistake conviviality for competence, cooptation for cooperation.

Some managed mental health firms, not the majority, are organized as staff models. They employ their own practitioners and in effect blend two roles—provider and manager of care. The dependency issue here may be a somewhat more difficult one; as employees, mental health professionals are likely to be more financially dependent upon their employer than are independent practitioners on any single referral source. To be certain that their professional judgments are not unduly influenced by what they perceive to be the needs of the organizations for which they work, it is important for these staff model firms to monitor the performance of their staff members. The contexts in which they work do affect their perceptions, beliefs and behavior and can overcome the professional identification to which I referred earlier.

There does appear to be at least anecdotal evidence suggesting that inpatient utilization levels in mental health services managed by staff model firms are lower than in others. Whether and to what extent this is true and if so, why, are important questions, the answers to which could influence the way managed mental health develops.

This is not to suggest that those managed mental health firms who work with independent practitioners do not also need to be concerned about the danger of unintentionally coopting their own staff. They also employ mental health professionals, not as providers but as care managers who influence the amount and type of services provided. They must be alert to the possibility that their care managers are also influenced by the ethos in which they work and could make decisions about patient care that may be unduly restrictive. Clinical case conferences, ongoing supervision, case review, and an open discussion of these issues are all processes that can help.

I discussed earlier the threats to quality that could result from the growth and increased competition between managed mental health firms if they are not sensitive to these issues. It is much less difficult to alter the delicate balance between managing care wisely and inappropriately withholding it than it is to recognize that it is happening. Managed mental health operates in an environment in which providers and care managers have broad discretion and freedom of judgment. And discretion is at the root of moral dilemmas: where there is no discretion there are few moral problems.

With growth and power comes responsibility. As we head into the last decade of this century, those of us in managed mental health must be careful not to transform our patients needs into our interests; their problems into our solutions; their insurance benefits into our programs. While we must be mindful of the warning by Samuel Butler that "The foundations of morality are like all other foundations; if you dig too much, the superstructure will come tumbling down" (Feldman, 1983), dig we must if managed mental health is to have a profound and positive effect on mental health services in what remains of the twentieth century and beyond.

REFERENCES

Bacon, K.H.: Private drug abuse treatment centers try to adjust to life in the slow lane. *Wall Street Journal,* 1990.

Berkman, L.: Hospital firm shows it's not afraid of risks. *Los Angeles Times,* 1991.

Broskowski, A.: Current mental health care environments: Why managed care is necessary. *Professional Psychology: Research and Practice, 22:*1, 1991.

Cost containment measures impede patient care. *Psychiatric News,* 1989.

England, M.J.: As quoted in: Popularity of managed care growing among insurers. *Psychiatric News,* 1989.

Feldman, S.: Conflict and convergence: The mental health professional in government. *Public Administration Review,* 1978.

Feldman, S.: Out of the hospital, onto the streets: The overselling of benevolence. *Hastings Center Report,* 1983.

Higgins, A.F.: *Health Care Benefits Survey:* Report #5. Princeton, N.J., 1990.

Kirshner, E.: Woes mount for addiction services firms as Parkside Med shuts down half of its centers. *Healthweek,* 1990.

Levinson, D.J. and Klerman, G.C.: The clinician-executive revisited. *Administration in Mental Health,* 1972.

Michels, R.: Psychoanalysis: The second century. *Harvard Mental Health Letter,* 1990.

Open Minds: More states pass utilization review laws. 3:2, 1990.

Raelin, J.: *The Clash of Cultures.* Boston: Harvard Business School Press, 1986.

Relman, A.: Assessment and accountability. *New England Journal of Medicine, 319:*18, 1988.

Trustees attack managed care threat. *Psychiatric News,* 1990.

Zimet, C.: The mental health care revolution: Will psychologists survive? *American Psychologist, 44:*4, 1989.

Chapter 2

MANAGED MENTAL HEALTH AND GROUP HEALTH INSURANCE

Michael J. Goran

The group health insurance industry is in the process of reforming itself once again to demonstrate that competition can constrain rising health costs. Despite the substantial growth of managed care, health insurance premiums for all employees have continued to rise. Many employers and policy makers are becoming frustrated with multiple choice and are beginning to question the cost containment potential of managed fee-for-service, health maintenance organizations (HMOs) and preferred provider organizations (PPOs).

If competition does not contain costs, the most likely alternative is for a stronger government role and a program similar to the one in Canada. A number of policy makers do not believe that competition has had an adequate test. They question whether employers have either fully committed to competition or understand the theory well enough to manage it properly. Enthoven (1989) suggests that "managed competition," which requires a much more sophisticated approach by employers, can work to contain costs and perform much better than the current multiple choice approach (Jones, 1989).

The group insurance industry is also working to demonstrate the cost containment potential of aggressive forms of managed care and "managed competition." A number of observers believe there will continue to be consolidation within the industry. Successful group health insurers will have to expand their efforts to become managers of health care delivery systems in addition to providing traditional insurance and administrative services.

The leading group health insurance companies (including Prudential, Travelers, CIGNA, Aetna, Metropolitan and a number of Blue Cross plans) are trying to shift more of the market into aggressive managed care benefit plans. These plans generally require beneficiaries to select a responsible primary care case manager and use a specific provider network. With these aggressive managed care plans, group health insurers believe the rise in health care costs can be constrained.

The leading HMOs (including Kaiser, U.S. Healthcare, and United HealthCare) continue to show strong growth. There is a widespread belief that the key to containing costs is to shift more of the market into HMO-type delivery systems because of their ability to better control the use of services and the rate of payment to providers while maintaining and, perhaps, ultimately improving the quality of care. Group health insurers and HMOs are marketing HMO-type delivery systems that offer point-of-service choice and cost sharing to employees with incentive/risk sharing to employers. In either case, these systems are capable of replacing the standard insurance plan.

A point-of-service plan provides incentives in the form of reduced costs and increased benefits to use a specified network of providers. Non-network providers may be used but there are financial disincentives to do so, usually a co-insurance and/or a deductible. Point-of-service plans are like PPOs in that non-network providers can be chosen but at reduced benefits. Unlike most PPOs, however, point-of-service plans are based on HMO-like delivery systems; they are sometimes called open-ended HMOs.

Mental health insurance and the mental health/substance abuse delivery systems are increasingly affected by these changes. The costs of mental health services are rising faster than general health. Yet, some employers are concerned that HMOs, in their efforts to contain expenses, are making it too difficult to obtain access to certain types of medically necessary mental health and substance abuse services. The current mental health system is vulnerable. As general health insurance shifts to aggressive managed care, mental health will either be provided as part of a broad managed care plan or "carved out" as a separate managed mental health network. Regardless of the direction, the current fee-for-service system is changing. Furthermore, if mental health expenses are not constrained, employers could resort to benefit cuts.

Over 10% of the health care dollar is now spent on mental health and substance abuse, and the proportion is growing. For some employers, mental health now accounts for over 20% of expenditures. Some of the increase represents greater demand, but there is growing concern that more services do not necessarily result in improved mental health. To contain these costs, a number of payors are attempting to manage their mental health and substance abuse programs. Managed care includes a range of techniques designed to control the cost and utilization of services, from managed fee-for-service (e.g., preadmission certification review) to the use of limited provider networks found in PPOs and HMOs. In mental health, the most common managed care arrangements are:

1. Specialized utilization review
2. Specialized mental health and substance abuse provider networks
3. Specialized case management

To understand the potential impact of managed care on the mental health system, one must first understand the changes that are taking place in general health insurance as it evolves to managed care. While there are special considerations regarding mental health and substance abuse services, mental health must co-exist with and, to an increasing extent, even depend on the general medical and surgical care delivery and financing environment.

The Changing Health Insurance Environment

In 1988, employer-sponsored health insurance protected 160 million Americans against the cost of illness. The Health Insurance Association of America (HIAA) estimates that more than 70% of Americans with employer-sponsored coverage are now enrolled in a managed care plan (Gabel, et al 1989). Most are in managed fee-for-service (43%) but 18% belong to HMOs and 11% to PPOs. Enrollment in pure HMOs (not point-of-service or open-ended) reached 32.5 million in July 1989; but, the rate of growth slowed and the number of HMOs declined.

In the mid-1980s, HMOs experienced rapid growth. There were substantial increases in their enrollment and number. In 1983, there were fewer than 14 million members in 290 HMOs. Enrollment grew to 21 million in 1985, 25.8 million in 1986, and 30.3 million in 1988. The number of HMOs peaked at 653 in 1988. The decline in the number of HMOs from 607 to 590 between January 1, 1989 and July 1, 1989 was due to several mergers and 12 terminations (Interstudy 1989). By the late 1980s, a number of them began to experience financial difficulties. Currently, HMOs are concentrating on controlled growth and are experiencing improved financial performance.

Group health insurers experienced annual rates of medical cost inflation in excess of 20% in 1988 and 1989. The HIAA Survey (which, because it excludes federal employees and individuals insured through a union or professional group, is probably conservative) found that health insurance premiums rose 12% between 1987 and 1988, nearly double the rate of increase from 1986 to 1987. From 1987 to 1988 two-thirds of all firms experienced rate increases. Those with standard health insurance plans increased an average of 20%, PPOs increased 27% and HMO premiums from 10% to 11%. The average monthly cost of health insurance in 1988 was approximately $100 for an individual and more than $200 for family coverage.

Health care spending now consumes nearly 12% of this country's gross national product. Overall spending has been growing rapidly and the Department of Commerce projects that it will continue to do so at a rate of 10% to 14% annually for the next five years (U.S. Industry Outlook, 1989). .

Those firms in the private sector that must also account for retiree health care costs have an additional strain on expenses. A decision by the Financial Accounting Standards Board requires that employers reflect as liabilities on their balance sheets the amount of health care benefits promised to retirees. This change is expected to add billions to their financial obligations. At the same time, about 35 million Americans are underinsured or have no health insurance. Health care cost containment has become a strategic imperative for private employers and government.

There is growing evidence that the increases in health care costs are due, in part, to our inefficient system. Other factors often mentioned (e.g., technology, defensive medicine and the aging population) only account for a part of the increased costs. While quality of care is becoming more important to purchasers and patients, there is little evidence to prove that our increased expenditures are buying more value. Wide variations still exist in the frequency of surgical procedures from one community to another. Many hospitals continue to perform complex surgical procedures in very low volume and, as a result, surgical teams do not have enough experience to maintain expertise. "Centers of Excellence" programs are being established by a number of insurers and employers to concentrate certain types of tertiary care (e.g., transplants) in a select group of facilities where volumes are high and excellent outcomes have been demonstrated.

The rise in health care costs is attributable to a number of factors other than inefficiency and general inflation. These include:

An aging population

Over the next 30 years, the population 65 years or older will reach 17% (compared with 12% in 1990). By the year 2020, there will be 50 million people over 65, almost half of them over 75, and seven million over 85. The elderly consume from two and one-half to four times the health care services of the under 65 population.

New technology

Constantly changing and rapidly growing, new technology includes neonatal intensive care at $1500 a day, complex infertility technology at $10,000 for a trial of in vitro fertilization, a $1,000 neogenetic resonance imaging procedure and multiple organ transplants that cost hundreds of thousands of dollars. Many new technologies are life-saving; nearly all require the extensive involvement of expert technicians and of physicians. Unfortunately, many new technologies supplement rather than replace existing ones. Some of the new ones such as neonatal intensive care and organ transplants raise complex ethical and legal questions.

Defensive medicine

Numerous tests and procedures are performed when clinical indications are soft but they are ordered anyway to protect the physician from subsequent litigation. A typical example is ordering a skull x-ray and a CAT scan for a child who has sustained relatively minor head trauma and has no immediate indications of neurologic damage. Another example is the use of fetal monitoring even though clinical indications are absent or minimal.

Increased use of out-patient hospital services and of specialized diagnostic tests and procedures

Radiation therapy and chemotherapy, invasive cardiology, arthroscopy, sophisticated new ways to use laser surgery, and lithotripsy are examples of specialized outpatient services and procedures.

Increased use of inpatient mental health services for adolescents

The availability of facilities and clinicians specializing in the diagnosis and treatment of adolescents results in the increased use of lengthy inpatient care that would otherwise have been provided with less sophistication, intensity, and cost in an earlier era. Adolescent admissions to inpatient facilities increased from 118 to 153 per 100,000 from 1980–1986 even though the total adolescent population in the nation decreased by 11 percent (Psychiatric News, 1989).

Increased use of expensive pharmaceuticals

TPA for the treatment of coronary arterial stenosis and AZT for those with AIDS are well known examples of this. No doubt, others will be coming along, and at a rapid pace.

Cost shifting from the public to private sector

As Medicare contains its expenditures for inpatient hospital services by using a DRG payment system, hospitals substantially increase rates to the remaining payors who still pay charges. They also develop ways to unbundle and increase revenues for outpatient services. Physicians also begin to unbundle services as more payors move away from usual and customary reimbursement. Medicare's introduction of a relative value scale for paying providers is likely to exacerbate cost shifting. Ironically, a number of HMOs now find that they are paying more for an outpatient surgical procedure than for a one day stay in the hospital.

Growth of Managed Care

By 1988, the majority of Americans covered under an employer-sponsored plan were in some form of managed care, though most were in a relatively moderate form of managed fee-for-service. More aggressive forms of managed care involve the use of a specific provider network designed and administered to control the quality, cost and use of services. Managed fee-for-service includes the application of one or more of a variety of techniques to assure the medical necessity of services. These include precertification of in and outpatient hospital services and other expensive diagnostic and therapeutic procedures, concurrent review of hospital services with discharge planning, second opinion programs, retrospective review of ambulatory services and patterns of care, and case management of complex patients whose care is expensive and who may benefit from the waiver of customary coverage limits. In 1988, 65% of those covered by health insurance were required to participate in preadmission certification review to obtain full benefits, an increase of more than 20% over 1987 (Gabel et al., 1989).

The growth of managed care has been dramatic. In 1980, only 4% of those covered by group health insurance were enrolled in an HMO or PPO. Today, more than 30% are. Alex Brown and Sons (1989) projects that up to 75% of the market could be in aggressive managed care programs within five years. This means that most of those now in managed fee-for-service plans will convert to an HMO, point-of-service plan or a more traditional PPO.

Managed fee-for-service has grown rapidly as commercial insurers and the Blues have attempted to introduce cost containment into their traditional plans to constrain premium increases and maintain benefits. Most employers have been receptive to adding moderate forms of managed care to their standard insurance plans in order to contain costs. This intermediate step allowed them to avoid more drastic alternatives such as dropping their standard plan altogether and only offering a choice of HMOs or PPOs (as has been done in a few areas such as Minneapolis-St. Paul).

In most instances, however, this initial move toward managed fee-for-service has not adequately contained costs. As a result, many employers are considering shifting to a more aggressive form of managed care or have already done so. Many observers believe that this shift will benefit a relatively small number of insurance companies and HMOs that have managed care capabilities in multiple locations and can take advantage of this growth to significantly increase the market share of their managed care products. Consolidations are likely to continue and a relatively small number of companies will emerge as managed care specialists.

Managed care companies are beginning to develop data on outcomes of care and other quality measures. Superior quality of care, patient satisfaction and information feedback to employers will emerge as a competitive advantage. If these new forms of managed care are able to contain costs, managed care companies will eventually compete more on quality and less on price and benefits.

Control of Costs

Premium increases appear to be continuing at about the same levels as in the past. With the majority of employer-covered Americans already in managed fee-for-service plans, one could argue that these moderate forms of managed care do not seem to be containing costs sufficiently.

What may be required is more aggressive forms of managed care like some HMOs where cost containment appears to be more effective.

In the last several years, payors have attempted to control costs with two approaches:

1. **Cost-shifting.** This approach produces savings for employers by shifting costs to the employee. It is done by adding deductibles and copayments and moving away from "first dollar" coverage. Employers can expect a decrease in the use and average cost of services when cost sharing is introduced. The Rand Study (Manning, et al, 1984) found that the introduction of even a five percent coinsurance for office visits (compared to no charge) substantially reduced the use of physician services. The concern is that if copayments become too high they will act as a deterrent to obtaining medically necessary services. Ultimately, cost-shifting has only a short-term potential because it is essentially a reduction in pay.

2. **Managed care.** Initially, this meant utilization review, preadmission certification, second surgical opinions, DRGs and encouraging employees to use alternative delivery systems. These techniques have had some success but not enough to contain the overall cost trend. Studies of utilization review found that total medical expenditures were reduced by about eight percent after controlling for employee and market characteristics and benefit plan features (Feldstein, et al, 1988). Other studies have found that the savings were reduced by shifts in the utilization of and expenditures on outpatient services (Custer, 1989).

Managed care has continued to evolve and many employers believe that the new, more sophisticated approaches hold promise for containing costs. Preadmission certification, for example, is being expanded to assure not only the medical necessity of elective hospital admissions, but also of ambulatory surgical procedures as well as expensive diagnostic procedures.

Preadmission screening uses criteria to determine the necessity of expensive procedures. Criteria sets are usually developed by expert clinicians, researchers and utilization review specialists and may be modified to fit local practice patterns. Reviewers, usually nurses, apply these criteria to individual cases. Patients or their physicians are asked to call an 800 number to obtain advance approval for services. If the cases meet the criteria, the nurse gives approval and frequently sets an estimated length of stay to initiate the concurrent review process if the services involve an inpatient stay. If the case under review does not meet the criteria or, as often happens, if it falls into an equivocal gray zone, a physician adviser is called in. The physician adviser is the only person who can deny preadmission approval. He discusses the case with the attending physician and makes a judgment call. The physician adviser may or may not have the same specialty as the attending physician, but is usually an experienced reviewer and has access to specialty reviewers if necessary.

Significant advances have been made in the quality, specificity and application of preadmission certification. Computer algorithms have been developed to screen the medical necessity of common procedures for in and outpatient care. These programs apply the results of sophisticated research to evaluating the quality of care and help to eliminate much of the equivocation about medical necessity.

Some firms have developed expertise in certain specialty areas as pharmaceuticals or mental health and substance abuse. A number of companies perform preadmission certification for psychiatric services using trained mental health clinicians. Most of these specialty firms get to know the practice patterns of local mental health providers and, over time, develop profiles of efficient practitioners and facilities. The specialty review firms also provide case management services. Case management procedures include early identification of potentially costly, complex cases and early intervention to ensure that the best available resources are provided. Case managers consult directly with the attending team and often provide valuable assistance in treatment planning. Case managers also often have the authority to waive benefit restrictions to make sure all steps are taken to reduce morbidity and overall costs.

Managed Care Networks

A number of health maintenance organizations have been able to contain costs and grow. Well-performing HMOs hold the most promise for controlling costs, in part, because they can be structured to reward efficiency. Group model HMOs such as Kaiser Permanente, have been able to keep their average annual premium increases much lower than those of the insurance industry. Although Kaiser's largest plan had a 19% increase in 1990, the average annual increase for the Company as a whole was less than 10% from 1980–1990. A few independent practice association (IPA) model plans have also contained costs, particularly those that rely on primary care case managers who receive capitation payments for patients in their panels. Capitation rewards them for containing specialty and hospital costs.

In the mid to late 1980s, a few PPOs began to perform like HMOs and evolved to become aggressive managed care companies. They developed sophisticated provider selection methods, information systems that produced comparative practice profiles, rigorous practice guidelines and state-of-the-art utilization control systems as well as financial incentives for efficient performance.

During the late 1980s, the distinctions between HMOs, PPOs, and managed fee-for-service began to blur. The leading group insurance carriers invested heavily in the development of managed care networks in most of the country's population centers. Prudential, CIGNA, Metropolitan, Aetna, and, in some markets, Blue Cross, all developed managed care networks in an attempt to combine the most cost-effective, employer-friendly features of HMOs, PPOs and managed fee-for-service. Other group insurers are either in the process of developing or expanding their own managed care networks (Travelers, New York Life, Lincoln, Principal, Private Care Initiative, CappCare) or getting out of the group health market (Transamerica, Allstate, Equicor).

Except for a few areas, employers are generally not comfortable enough with HMOs to offer a group or staff model and an IPA as the only health care benefit options (and give up the traditional indemnity plan). They are concerned that some of the HMO successes have been at the expense of the conventional indemnity plan because of adverse selection (where the "better" risks choose the HMO and the least healthy opt for indemnity coverage). They are also often concerned about the lack of adequate utilization and other information provided by HMOs and about the fairness of community rating (charging the same premium to employers regardless of the actual health care cost and utilization of their work force). Commercial insurance companies are more likely to set rates based on the actual experience of employees, particularly in large companies. As a result of pressure from employers and relaxation of the federal HMO law, many HMOs are beginning to move toward a modified form of experience rating known as adjusted community rating. Some employers are reducing the number of managed care plans they offer to lessen the administrative burden and reduce the risk of offering plans that may not be financially viable.

Employers are also concerned that employees and, where applicable, their unions will not accept a "lock-in" (in a traditional HMO plan there is no coverage for services that are obtained outside of the HMO, except for medical emergencies). They have been more willing to do so with mental health and substance abuse services. This is accomplished through an EPO (exclusive provider organization), a managed mental health provider network in which there is no coverage for services obtained out-of-network. The rationale for distinguishing between mental health and general medical services in this way includes:

- Costs of mental health and substance abuse are more out of control than general medical services
- Quality can be improved by requiring patients to use a selected mental health network, thereby eliminating the substantial variability in mental health practice patterns
- Employees and their families tend not to be concerned about a "lock-in" for mental health and substance abuse services (they do not generally perceive themselves as likely users of such services). Those who are using mental health services may be reluctant to complain openly to protect their privacy.

A number of large employers have come to realize that managed fee-for-service plans are not adequately containing costs as well as more aggressive approaches such as HMO-like managed care networks with point-of-service choice. They are adopting such networks and consolidating their health plan options even to a single point-of-service plan managed by one insurance carrier. Others are retaining a few HMOs in order to continue some competition between plans.

Point of Service

Sophisticated point-of-service (POS) plans are now offered by a number of insurance carriers and HMOs. They provide incentives (in the form of reduced costs and increased benefits) to use a specified network of providers. An out-of-network physician may be chosen but there is a financial disincentive to do so, in the form of higher deductibles and coinsurance. A typical plan might include an out-of-network deductible of $250, with a coinsurance of 30%. In-network benefits generally do not have a deductible and copayments are typically about $10 for an office visit.

When POS plans were first introduced, there was concern that people would resist changing physicians to maintain higher benefits levels. The assumptions were that out-of-network use would be very high and that there would be a lot of complaints about the added cost of using one's own non-network physician. Typical provider networks often include less than half, and frequently closer to one-quarter of the practicing physicians in a community. Though experience is still limited, the early POS plans are reporting both a high degree of acceptance and a relatively low proportion of out-of-network use.

The most important and aggressive feature of the POS is the replacement of the conventional unrestricted choice plan with a managed care network. The successful plans are likely to have all or most of the following characteristics:

- Multi-year guarantees (including some financial risk sharing) substantially lower than the projected costs of the conventional plan it is replacing
- The availability of provider networks that perform up to HMO standards and are geographically accessible
- Point-of-service choice for employees who do not wish to use network providers
- Risk-sharing arrangements between the program manager (usually an insurance carrier or an HMO) and the network providers
- Effective utilization management and comprehensive reporting of utilization and costs
- Use of primary care case management and, where possible, primary care capitation when networks are based on IPAs
- Capability to manage mental health and substance abuse costs
- Control of prescription drug costs
- Centers of excellence for complex tertiary care services
- Use of the managed care network to serve pre- and post-Medicare retirees
- Consolidation of other health plan options offered to employees (especially group or staff model HMOs) into a smaller number that will perform the best, have employee support, provide information and negotiate rates based on experience
- Use of employer contributions to force competition between the managed care network and the other plans.

Developing a Managed Care Strategy

Employers interested in cost containment must decide how aggressive they want to be. The fundamental trade-off is between cost containment and restrictions on employee freedom of choice. To help make the decision, employers first need to establish financial and human-resource objectives.

Financial objectives are best defined in an annual per capita cost target. To set a target and then determine how to reach it requires an understanding of baseline utilization, costs, and demographics. Employers need to know whether cost increases are more concentrated in specific geographic locations, or are attributable to certain services (e.g., mental health) or types of cases (e.g., catastrophic). By analyzing baseline experience and comparing it to the target objectives, employers will weigh the following options:

- Replace the conventional indemnity plan with a point-of-service managed care network and consolidate multiple choice offerings to a few well-performing competitive plans
- Be even more aggressive, eliminate the conventional plan and offer several HMOs in its place
- Maintain the conventional plan, but confine the employer contribution to the total premium in terms of the lowest-cost option available, most likely a group or staff model HMO

If the first option is selected, employers will likely go through a competitive bidding process to select a program manager to administer both the network and out-of-network portions of the plan. The program manager, typically an insurance carrier or an HMO, assumes administrative and financial responsibility for all of the employer's health care benefits except those provided by the HMOs that are retained as multiple choice offerings.

The competitive bidding process provides employers with a method to design a managed care network that meets their needs. At pre-bidders conferences with potential program managers, the employer shares financial, utilization, and demographic data and discusses needs and objectives. Bidders are requested to provide detailed information on a range of competitive features.

The program manager is typically selected after analyzing written proposals and site visits. Three factors are key to the selection process:

1. Adequacy of the network. Is there sufficient geographic coverage? Is the provider selection process rigorous enough? Is the mix of providers by specialty type adequate? What is the track record of the providers? Are the provider contracts designed to reward efficient behavior? Are the quality assurance and utilization control programs adequate?

2. Financial terms. Will the bidder accept risk and agree to a cost target? At what price? How much risk is the bidder willing to assume and for how long a period? Will the bidder share risk with the employer above and below a cost target?

3. Administrative capabilities. What are the costs for administering the managed care network plan? Does the bidder have sufficient experience? Does the bidder have an integrated claims system? Can the bidder report comprehensive information about utilization and costs? Is there capacity to produce practice profiles?

Implications for Mental Health

As more employers become aggressive about health care cost containment, the use of managed care networks will grow. The major issue for mental health and substance abuse services will not be how to avoid these changes but how best to cope with them. Employers will have to decide whether to keep mental health and substance abuse services within their general managed care network or to carve them out. If carved out, the services are delivered through a specialized provider network that should include utilization control, quality assurance measures, provider selection, and financial incentives appropriate to the mental health setting.

Mental health and substance abuse providers increasingly need to concern themselves with meeting the eligibility requirements of general and specialized managed care networks. They also need to become expert in providing quality mental health services within a primary care case managed environment.

An important consequence of the new managed care environment for mental health professionals and their patients is the growing reliance on the primary care physician as case manager or "gatekeeper." Most employers and insurers believe that committed primary care physicians are essential to controlling the use of the rest of the health care system. As a result, managed care plans often require that individuals select a primary care physician (PCP) who will also function as a case manager.

The approval of the PCP is required before consulting with a specialist such as a mental health professional. Frequently, benefits are reduced if such approval is not obtained.

This approach has serious implications for mental health. Many patients are accustomed to having direct access to a mental health professional. A referral from a PCP will be a new requirement for them. While many mental health professionals are accustomed to working with primary care and specialty physicians on a referral basis, the requirement of such a referral may well be viewed as a barrier to care. But the PCP is not merely supposed to screen patients to determine the necessity of referral to a mental health professional. In many managed care programs, the physician is expected to diagnose and treat common, uncomplicated mental disorders. The mental health professional may be asked to consult but the PCP will retain responsibility for treatment.

Some managed care programs do recognize the special nature of mental health services and allow direct access to them, bypassing the normal authorization requirements. If mental health cost and utilization trends continue at levels in excess of general medical trends, however, direct access is likely to be constrained.

Mental Health "Carve Out"

Many managed mental health programs permit direct access to mental health care. Because these "carve out" managed mental health programs appear better able to control costs, it is likely that direct access to them will continue, even as it is constrained in the general gatekeeper environment. The specialized "carved out" managed mental health and substance abuse network does appear to hold promise. A number of employers have endorsed the approach and specialized networks are growing at a rapid rate throughout the county. They appear to be taking seriously the need for cost-effective behavior by constraints on the autonomy of providers through the use of objective criteria, explicit treatment objectives and aggressive clinical management. Patients who would otherwise receive inpatient care followed by a lengthy course of outpatient treatment in the fee-for-service setting are being treated with alternatives to inpatient care such as short-term crisis intervention and goal-oriented outpatient therapy.

In the managed care environment, many of the decisions that were left to the discretion of the patient and/or the mental health professional become prerogatives of the managed care plan. A typical "carve out" mental health and substance abuse managed care plan has policies and procedures that address the following:

- Who to call when services are desired
- Who is responsible for the initial patient evaluation
- Whether clinicians who do the initial patient evaluations should be allowed to also treat the patient
- The use of cost-effective treatment such as brief outpatient psychotherapy and alternatives to inpatient care
- The role of non medical mental health professionals in the diagnosis and treatment of patients
- The role of group, family and other therapies
- The use of psychoactive medications
- Diagnosis and treatment of the seriously mentally ill
- Selection of and contracting with practitioners and facilities
- Treatment options for substance abuse and dual diagnosis
- Adolescent and child diagnosis and treatment options
- The relationship of the managed mental health program to the general medical plan
- Utilization and quality management
- Levels and methods of compensation for providers
- The degree and type of financial incentives/risk sharing

"Carve out" managed mental health programs attempt to maintain mental health benefits and contain or decrease costs by reducing the inappropriate use of inpatient services, and emphasizing brief outpatient treatment. Not all patients or therapists agree with this approach. The introduction of a managed mental health plan can be frustrating for mental health professionals and their patients. To ease the transition to a managed plan, mental health professionals must commit the time necessary to learn how to function best in a managed care environment. With the projected growth of such plans, this will be necessary if mental health professionals want to maintain continuity of care for existing patients and be accessible to new ones.

Change will continue in group health insurance. Most of the remaining traditional health insurance plans will be replaced by one form or another of managed care. This will require all health care providers, including those in mental health, to change their behavior and develop expertise in cost-effective diagnosis and treatment. Before long, it is likely that most mental health practitioners and facilities will be participating in general medical as well as specialized managed mental health programs.

REFERENCES

Cost containment measures will continue chokehold. *Psychiatric News, 24:*11, 1989.

Custer, W.S.: *Employer Health Care Plan Design, Plan Costs, and Health Care Delivery.* The Employee Benefit Research Institute, Washington, D.C., 1989.

Enthoven, A.C.: Effective management of competition in the FEBHP. *Health Affairs,* 1989.

Feldstein, P.J. et al.: Private cost containment, the effects of utilization review programs on health care use and expenditures. *New England Journal of Medicine,* 1310–1314, 1988.

Gabel, J., DiCarlo, S., Fink, S. and deLissovoy, G.: DataWatch: employer-sponsored health insurance in America. *Health Affairs,* 1989.

Group Health to Change Rapidly in the 1990s Providing Investment Opportunities. Alex Brown & Sons, Baltimore, Maryland, 1989.

Gruber, L., Shadle, M., and Pion, K.: HMO growth slowdown continues. *Interstudy Edge,* 1989.

Jones, S.B.: Perspective: can multiple choice be managed to constrain health care costs? *Health Affairs,* 1989.

Manning, W.G., et al.: A controlled trial of the effect of a prepaid group practice on use of services. *New England Journal of Medicine,* 1505–1510, 1984.

U.S. Department of Commerce: *U.S. Industry outlook.* 51-1-51-6, 1989.

Chapter 3

MANAGED MENTAL HEALTH IN THE PUBLIC SECTOR

Trevor R. Hadley, Arie Schinnar and Aileen Rothbard

Over the last 30 years, the public mental health system has used a variety of financing and management models to provide services. The recent emergence of managed care in the private general medical and mental health sectors has led to much discussion and some experimentation in the delivery of public mental health services (Mechanic and Aiken, 1989).

The concept of managed care has a long history in mental health. Prior to the deinstitutionalization movement of the 1960s and 1970s, most state psychiatric hospitals served as the care management system for public patients. A single entity, the state hospital provided both inpatient and ambulatory care services and made all staffing, financial, and program decisions.

The use of managed care in the outpatient public sector was an integral part of the community mental health center concept. Community mental health centers (CMHCs) were designed to provide comprehensive mental health services to a defined population (catchment area). They received federal and state funds to provide needed services to those areas. The early literature on the community mental health center movement assumed that the CMHCs were mandated to provide services to all those in need (Morrissey and Goldman, 1984). In the early 1960s, much energy, effort, and money were expended to design assessment tools in order to determine the need for various types of mental health services in each of the catchment areas and then to develop coordinated and managed systems to provide the appropriate care. These earlier concepts of a public sector managed mental health network for a defined geographic area are now being recreated by the public system managed care initiatives of the last several years.

Current Patterns of Care

The current public system is perceived by policymakers, funders, advocates and consumers as fragmented and inefficient. Much of the fragmentation is related to the development of new funding mechanisms that have fueled a dramatic expansion of the public mental health service system (Goering, Wasylenki, Farkas, Lancee and Ballantyne, 1988).

In addition to the development of CMHCs, Medicare and Medicaid have contributed to the growth but also to the fragmentation of the system. Medicaid and Medicare reimburse CMHCs, general hospitals and other facilities on a fee-for-service basis (Sharfstein, 1982). This reimbursement system helped create a new group of inpatient care providers. Acute care general hospital psychiatric units and an acute care "industry" developed across the country. With no limitation on the amount of care provided and no financial risk to the provider or patient, costs escalated and the system grew (Thompson, 1986). Despite this growth during the 1970s, state and local mental health authorities believed that the chronic mentally ill needed additional services. New programs such as the Community Support Program were created (Turner and Tenhoor, 1978). The focus on and increased funding for the needs of the severely and persistently mentally ill encouraged the establishment of new provider agencies offering such services as psychosocial and vocational rehabilitation and residential care. As a result, the nation-wide mental health service system now includes more than 5,000 organizations; over 3,500 of them receive some state government support (Lutterman, Mazade, Wurster, and Glover, 1988; Mandersheid and Barrett, 1987).

This expansion has provided substantially more care for public patients but has increased the fragmentation of the system. Today, one client may be involved with five or six different public sector service providers at the same time. While this increase in the number of providers made more services available, it added to the fragmentation, decreased continuity and exacerbated the clinical and financial management problems (Dorwart, 1988; Talbott, 1985).

These problems have led mental health policymakers to propose variants of managed care and capitation plans for the public sector (Lehman, 1987; Talbott and Sharfstein, 1986). These proposals are, in general, motivated by attempts to reduce the discontinuity and fragmentation of care. Government agencies such as Medicaid and Medicare, are concerned about the increasing cost of public mental health services and they see managed care as a potential cost containment measure.

CURRENT EXPERIMENTS AND DEMONSTRATIONS

Minnesota

A number of state and local mental health agencies are experimenting with various capitation approaches to financing and organizing mental health services. These experiments include at least four different approaches to capitation as the vehicle of managed care. The first includes mental health services as part of general health capitation programs using public funds. A project in Minnesota involved the mandatory enrollment in health maintenance organizations (HMOs) of Medicaid clients in two counties and a portion of the city of Minneapolis (Christianson, Lurie, Finch and Moscovice, 1988). Begun in 1985, this program shifted the control of mental health services from the county mental health authorities to HMOs under contract with the state. All health and mental health services previously reimbursed by Medicaid on a fee-for-service basis were provided by the HMOs with some special provisions for the chronic mentally ill. The HMOs were paid a predetermined contractual amount.

Many of the public mental health providers were concerned about the program. They worried that the HMOs were inexperienced with the seriously mentally ill and that the disincentives to provide services in a capitated system might result in underutilization by this particularly vulnerable population. They were also concerned about a reduction in Medicaid revenue to their agencies. The program's effect on the providers, however, was quite small as most clients continued with their prior public sector agencies.

The HMOs had reservations about including the chronic mentally ill in the demonstration. In the beginning, they were concerned about providing social rather than medical services. Later on, a number of them believed they were seeing too many of the seriously mentally ill. In 1987, some of the HMOs began to experience serious financial difficulties as a result of high use of their services by Aid to Families with Dependent Children (AFDC) recipients. State officials dropped the disabled Medicaid eligible group (blind and/or disabled recipients) from the demonstration in order to ensure its continuation (Christianson,

Lurie, Finch, and Moscovice, 1989). This removed most of the mentally ill. Evaluation of the demonstration is ongoing.

South Carolina

In South Carolina, a joint project between the Department of Mental Health and the Medicaid program is using a similar model to voluntarily enroll Medicaid eligible recipients in a capitation plan that covers all health and mental health services for the chronic mentally ill. The Department of Mental Health has contracted with CMHCs to manage and coordinate the health and mental health services (South Carolina, 1987). The project allows the Medicaid recipients to choose their health care providers, but restricts their mental health care to the CMHCs. The Department of Mental Health is using a capitation system to finance outpatient mental health services and a portion of the state hospital costs. Other hospital psychiatric and general health care will be funded through Medicaid. This project differs from the one in Minnesota in that it maintains existing client/mental health center relationships.

Philadelphia

Another capitated model funds only public sector mental health services. One such model was developed in Philadelphia by the Robert Wood Johnson Foundation and the U.S. Department of Housing and Urban Development Initiative for the Chronically Mentally Ill. It was designed to encourage the development of innovative ways to provide mental health care to the growing chronic mentally ill (CMI) population. Philadelphia was one of nine cities chosen to serve as demonstration sites (Aiken, Somers and Shore, 1986). At each site, the program intends to create an organizational structure that combines administrative, fiscal and service responsibility for providing care to the chronic mentally ill; to develop community-wide systems of care offering a broad range of health, mental health, social services and housing options for them; to assist the chronic mentally ill to function more effectively in their everyday lives; and to strengthen their potential to live independently (Aiken, Somers and Shore, 1986).

The Philadelphia plan seeks to implement these objectives through three major changes in the provision of services (Rothbard, Hadley and Schinnar, 1989). Divergent funding streams will be consolidated under one central authority. This will include existing county mental health funds, Medicaid reimbursement paid directly to provider agencies, and state funds currently supporting state psychiatric hospital beds for Philadelphia. The goal is to provide flexibility in the use of program resources in order to encourage the use of less expensive ambulatory instead of more costly inpatient care. Theoretically, this should reduce the overall cost of inpatient services and expand the resources available for ambulatory care. The City will introduce several changes at the service provision level: (1) intensive case management for heavy utilizers of services; (2) selection of preferred providers for inpatient care; (3) a process of preadmission screening and length of stay reviews; (4) performance contracts to the local mental health centers and (5) new residential beds to provide long-term care for the chronic mentally ill. The focus of the experiment is on developing interventions designed to deal specifically with high utilizers of inpatient care who are not well served by the current ambulatory care system (Hadley, Schinner, Rothbard and Kinosian, 1989).

Although this project has been slowed somewhat by changes in administration, several phases are now under way. The central authority is in place and is responsible for the heavy user case management program. The consolidation of state psychiatric hospital funds will be completed by the end of 1990 and Medicaid funds are now capitated for inpatient care in a portion of the city.

New York

The third public sector approach to managed care through capitation puts a contracting provider at risk for the care. In this model, a high-risk subgroup of mental health clients is usually identified by disability or prior utilization. The responsibility for providing care is contracted to a provider or group of providers on an at-risk basis. In the Monroe/ Livingston area of New York State, a capitated system began operation in 1987 (Babigian and Marshall, 1989). A non-profit corporation functions as the manager of a number of funding streams that are combined to make single capitation payments possible. Subsets of chronic mentally ill patients have been assigned to one of three risk groups on the basis of different historical levels of service utilization (Babigian and Reed, 1986). The groups are: continuous ($39,000/year), intermittent ($13,000/ year), and outpatient ($5,000/year).

The corporation contracts for the care of eligible patients. The contracted providers deliver outpatient care and are responsible for state hospital utilization by their patients. The project has focused on the state hospital population, but is expanding to include patients with similar levels of disability without much prior state hospital experience. The primary goal is to provide financial incentives to expand outpatient and residential services for the chronic mentally ill and reduce the use of long-term inpatient care at the state hospital. Early results indicate an initial reduction of inpatient care and a relatively dramatic increase in outpatient services provided to these clients (Babigian and Marshall, 1989).

The New York State Office of Mental Health has begun experimenting with the use of capitated arrangements to pay for specific services (Surles and Blanch, 1989). In one demonstration, the state is funding an intensive case management program characterized by extremely aggressive aftercare programs, small case loads, and emergency access. In some areas, the program is funded on a capitated basis and in others through fee-for-service. The state will evaluate the impact of these financial arrangements on service utilization, cost and clinical outcomes.

Rhode Island

A fourth model provides an individual capitation payment to a provider. To decrease the population in particular state psychiatric hospitals, a state assigns a bounty or number of dollars to a particular patient or group of patients. The payment is offered ·as a capitated fee to provide services to that individual or group outside the state hospital. Rhode Island pioneered this approach in 1982 when it gave additional funds to local community providers to move clients out of state hospitals. The state was able to substantially reduce the hospital census (Mauch, 1989).

In 1987, Rhode Island began a second phase of this project. The payments are tied to specific patients who have been assigned to two risk categories: Transfer I clients (need outpatient support and independent living assistance) and Transfer II clients (are more disabled and need long-term care and substantial support). These payments are provided in addition to the routine ones to community providers and to the reimbursements received from third party payors. Transfer I, begun in 1982, included 210 clients. The decreased state hospital utilization of these clients resulted in a 70–80 reduction in hospital beds—all 210 clients are living in the community instead of the hospital. Transfer II, where the payment was almost four times the level of Transfer I, has resulted in an additional decrease of approximately 80 beds.

The objective in all these experiments is to encourage the substitution of less for more intensive services. Past financial strategies, dependent on medical reimbursement systems such as Medicare and Medicaid, encouraged hospital-based care. Many of the managed care/capitation demonstrations are interested in the development of services such as case management and psychosocial rehabilitation as alternatives to the use of acute and long-term psychiatric beds. Without the development and use of managed care/capitation to replace the widespread fee-for-service system, the substitution of alternatives to hospital care cannot occur.

In general, experiments with capitation approaches to managed care in the public sector are designed to provide better coordination of services and to discourage the use of inpatient care. Under managed care, incentives can be designed to provide more effective individualized treatment, particularly for the chronic mentally ill. Most proposals attempt to accomplish this by combining a variety of diverse public sector funding streams and transferring some of the financial risk to local authorities and/or providers responsible for rendering and coordinating community based services. Regulatory controls ordinarily imposed by the different funding agencies would be relaxed to allow for increased flexibility. Centralized clinical management, coordination and oversight of the services provided are, at least theoretically, combined with a decentralized community based mental health system.

Opportunities and Risks

The provision of mental health services through capitated financing mechanisms requires the development of a single funding stream. Diverse sources of funds must be consolidated under a single authority in order to support a wide array of patient services. This authority may be a county, a community center or a private health management organization under contract to a public agency. It will coordinate all of the services for which the targeted population is eligible. Eligibility may be based on geography, income and employment as well as on severity and chronicity of illness. This arrangement simplifies the otherwise typical arrangement in which a patient receiving publicly financed services may have inpatient care funded by Medicare, day treatment by Medicaid and psychosocial rehabilitation services by the local mental health authority.

Capitation with single stream funding requires a reorganization of services under an administrative body capable of allocating an entire bundle of resources to provide those services that best meet the needs of an eligible client population. It also entails an inter-organizational transfer of resources between state, federal, and local agencies, as well as private enterprises. The resource transfer is often accompanied by a transfer of responsibility for patient care and the financial risk associated with that care. The transfer of responsibility and risk may follow two paths, a top-down or "downstream" funding approach or a bottoms-up "upstream" one.

In a downstream capitation plan, funds are transferred from federal and state government to local authorities such as the county or to individual community providers. Downstream capitation financing provides opportunities for state legislators to contain spiraling mental health costs, make better predictions for future budgets, and transfer financial responsibility and risk to local authorities (Christianson, 1987). While they may also seek to transfer political responsibility for the mental health services, such transfers are extremely difficult to achieve since ultimately the responsibility rests with them. The local school board is an example of the downstream approach.

An upstream capitation plan entails a transfer of service provision responsibility from the local providers to a higher level such as a county or state government. An example of such a plan would be the consolidation of different inpatient and outpatient providers under one organizational umbrella—a government or private not-for-profit organization. Under such a reorganization, the local providers transfer financial authority and accountability while the central authority assumes primary responsibility for overall program planning.

Although financial risks may flow either up or down the organizational ladder, the political risk and responsibility always remain at the top. But the responsibility and risk associated with patient treatment always remain at the bottom, at the provider level. Under a downstream capitation plan, the political authority loses its financial flexibility and is less able to respond to political changes. The result is an increase in political risk, while downstream providers gain flexibility in reallocating resources to better serve the client population (Schinnar, Rothbard, and Hadley, 1989).

In an upstream capitation plan, providers lose control over the financial resources, thereby decreasing their ability to be more responsive to patient needs. Provider risk associated with patient care ultimately increases under this scenario. The top of the organization, however, is strengthened as political factors can be more easily translated into funding priorities. Special interest groups also gain potency in an upstream model although they still must compete with others. In this environment, policy priorities rather than individual patient needs form the basis for patient care.

The downstream model gives greater authority to individual providers in setting treatment priorities and meeting patient needs. Most public system experiments are downstream like the Philadelphia plan. The upstream models are more typical of the private health sector where individual physicians are grouped into HMO, PPO, or IPA arrangements.

Substitution and Continuity of Services

The principal effect of a capitation financing design with single stream funding is flexibility in resource allocation. A primary goal is to achieve substitution of community-based services for more costly inpatient care. If successful, substitution should provide resources for the development of innovative community-based programs (Lehman, 1987). One major assumption is at least implicit in any plan for substitution of services— that the demand for outpatient care is not sated and that by increasing the intensity of outpatient services and case management, hospital utilization (admissions and lengths of stay) will be significantly reduced. Since many users of inpatient services resist outpatient care, however, substitution may not be effective for all patient populations (the elderly, for example).

A reduction in length of stay achieved through increased utilization of ambulatory care may also result in higher readmission rates. This is especially true if intensive case management programs that provide increased continuity of care are introduced as part of the capitation plan. Thus, it is not clear that substitution of alternatives to inpatient care will achieve any significant savings, particularly when the emergency room is used frequently by the chronic patient population (Surles and McGurrin, 1987) and is therefore an appropriate site for case management. Substitution of ambulatory for inpatient services may be effectively accomplished when a case manager is aware of the emergency room visit and arranges for a referral to ambulatory rather than inpatient care. If the patient in crisis tends primarily to be a user of emergency room services followed only rarely by hospitalization, the intervention of case management will increase the use of outpatient services and may actually bring about increased inpatient use, thereby increasing the overall cost of care for these patients (Goering, Wasylenki, Farkas, Lancee and Ballantyne, 1988). Early findings from the evaluations of a number of intensive case management projects lend support to this judgment (Franklin, Solovitz, Mason and Clemons, 1987; Worley, 1989). This may, however, be only a short-term effect.

In Philadelphia, turnover rates for a treated Medicaid population are estimated to be about 30% per annum. Over a two-year period, only 40% of the Medicaid population received services in two consecutive years (Hadley, 1990; Hadley, McGurrin, Schinnar and Rothbard, 1988). If case management significantly increases continuity of care and thus moderates patient turnover, annual enrollment in public mental health programs and therefore their costs, may increase.

Cost Shifts and "Spillover" Effects

Since downstream capitation involves a transfer of financial risk from state and federal government to local authorities, the management of capitation plans may be fiscally conservative. To minimize financial risk, the plan manager will invariably focus attention on the more costly users of the mental health system. They are likely to be targeted for special case management interventions as in Philadelphia and New York. These interventions will generally be manifested by performance contracts to local providers or financial incentives attached to performance and cost saving measures. While such strategies may be cost effective for the population and programs under the capitation plan, a variety of "spillover" effects and cost shifting may limit the overall success of the plan.

Targeting high service users for priority care may crowd out moderate users, especially when resources are scarce. This may result in a deterioration in the mental health status of the moderate users and subsequent increases in the long term cost of patients who do not receive appropriate care. Furthermore, if capitation is targeted to Medicaid eligible patients, as it often is, cost shifts may occur as community programs that are funded by local resources shift the cost of high risk patients from the capitation financed activities to others. This would be in direct response to system-wide incentives that are instituted to reduce the cost of high-risk patients. Nearly all such patients are found among the Medicaid population (Schinnar, Hadley and Rothbard, 1988).

Other possible cost shifts entail a change in locus of care from the mental health to the general health care system, especially for the elderly. It is generally believed that elderly patients are underserved in outpatient and other community-based mental health programs and tend to use hospital services when they do seek psychiatric care (Gottlieb and Bloom, 1987). If their access to psychiatric inpatient care is reduced as a result of capitation financing, their service needs may be met through the general health care system. In addition, shifts may occur from the acute care sector to step down or residential programs where the latter are funded or subsidized by federal dollars.

Organizational Economies and Staffing Changes

Downstream capitation funding brings about significant changes in the organization of mental health care. First and most significant is the reduction in choice of providers for the client population. This creates a distinction between the poor who are usually the recipients of mental health care under a publicly financed capitated system and the rest of the population. It is a major reversal of the original intent of the Medicaid and Medicare programs: to provide equity and access to care for all (Mechanic and Aiken, 1987). Although the fee-for-service Medicaid programs are often viewed as a source of discontinuity in the community mental health system and of bias toward inpatient services, they have afforded the poor and the elderly a wider array of quality psychiatric services otherwise not available to them (Schlesinger, 1989).

Managed care under capitation will tend to consolidate the number of current providers into a subset of "preferred providers." With approximately the same volume of patients served by fewer sites, the size of the programs per site is likely to increase. As this happens, will the cost per unit of service rise or fall? This will depend on whether economies of scale exist or are possible in the current system.

The introduction of new programs such as residential step down units, and intensive case management may not affect marginal costs significantly enough to reduce the average cost of care. If their introduction also entails substantial fixed costs, however, the result may be average costs that substantially exceed the marginal ones. This suggests that cost savings achieved through substitution of community-based services for inpatient care may be absorbed by high fixed costs associated with new programs. Whatever savings are achieved through service substitutions, need to be significant enough to cover both the fixed and variable cost of the new initiatives (Schinnar and Rothbard, 1989). When financial resources are transferred down, significant administrative costs are associated with new responsibilities. The indirect cost of such management must be included with any transfer of program funding in a downstream model.

Other cost concerns are associated with potential changes in staffing. Increased reliance on community-based programs under downstream capitation may require more psychiatric time, e.g., the severity of mental illness in the community population may increase as the use of acute hospital care services is reduced. Better qualified clinicians for intensive case management programs will be needed to provide clinical treatment as well as coordination and monitoring of patient care.

With all these risks, why is downstream capitation gaining acceptance? Largely because of the consensus that the current level of fiscal and administrative fragmentation is untenable (Bachrach, 1981; Mechanic and Aiken, 1987; Lehman, 1987; Talbott, 1986) and that the opportunity to substitute approaches other than repeated, extended inpatient stays is great.

Conclusion

In recent years, capitation has emerged as a mechanism for financing and managing mental health care. It is believed by some to be the answer to problems of fragmentation as well as to reducing or at least controlling escalating costs. Historically, most private capitated health plans have served the relatively young and employable low-risk populations. In the last decade, the idea of capitation as a mechanism for managing general medical services for high-risk groups, such as Medicare and Medicaid populations, has received increased attention.

Currently, capitation is being proposed by various authorities as a way to provide mental health care for the chronic mentally ill (Lehman, 1987). Proponents suggest that capitation will increase service flexibility, particularly in ambulatory services; offer new configurations of service that are broader, better coordinated, and less redundant; and encourage earlier intervention by reducing financial barriers to patients (Schlesinger, 1986). A system that integrates services under a single agency and provides patients with a case manager to guide them would facilitate appropriate and cost-effective care (Surles and Blanch, 1989).

Despite the proliferation of experiments with public sector capitated systems, it is too early to draw conclusions as to the best model. The range of current experiments with a variety of different models will, however, lead in the near future to a much better understanding of how capitation may operate effectively in the public system. It clearly offers options for service substitution and for the development of alternative service systems that are not possible in the current deficit funded and fee-for-service mixed model. It is also clear from the current experiments that unlike the insurance based mental health plans, the diversity and complexity of the funding for public mental health services argue not for a single capitation model but for a number of models specific to the resources, needs and constraints of the environments in which they will be implemented.

REFERENCES

Aiken, L.H., Somers, S.A., and Shore, M.F.: Private foundations in health affairs: A case study of the development of a national initiative for chronically mentally ill. *American Psychologist, 41:*1290–1295, 1986.

Babigian, H.M., and Marshall, P.E.: A comprehensive capitation experiment. In Mechanic, D. and Aiken, L. (Eds.): *Paying for Services: Promises and Pitfalls of Capitation* (New Directions for Mental Health Services Series). San Francisco, Jossey-Bass, 1989, vol 43, pp. 43–54.

Babigian, H.M., and Reed, S.K. *Integrated Mental Health: A Demonstration Project in Upstate New York.* New Haven, CT: Workshop on Developing a Research Agenda for Studying the Administration of Mental Health Services, 1986.

Bachrach, L.L.: Continuity of care for chronic mental patients: A conceptual analysis. *American Journal of Psychiatry, 138:* 1449–1456, 1981.

Christianson, J.B.: *A Comparative Study of Public Sector Capitated Financing Arrangements in Mental Health.* Washington, D.C., NASMHPD report under NIMH contract, 1987.

Christianson, J.B., Lurie, N., Finch, M., and Moscovice, I.: Mandatory enrollment of Medicaid-eligible mentally ill persons in prepaid health plans: The Minnesota demonstration project. *Administration and Policy in Mental Health, 16*(2):51–64, 1988.

Christianson, J.B., Lurie, N., Finch, M. and Moscovice, I.: Mainstreaming the mentally ill in HMO's. In Mechanic, D. and Aiken, L. (Eds.): *Paying for Services: Promises and Pitfalls of Capitation* (New Directions for Mental health Services Series), San Francisco: Jossey-Bass, 1989, vol. 43, pp. 19–28.

City of Philadelphia Application for Robert Wood Johnson Program for the Chronic Mentally Ill. Philadelphia, May 1986.

Dorwart, R.A.: A ten-year follow-up study of the effects of deinstitutionalization. *Hospital and Community Psychiatry, 39:*287–291, 1988.

Franklin, J., Solovitz, B., Mason, M., Clemons, J., and Miller, G.: An evaluation of case management. *American Journal of Public Health, 77*(6):674–678, 1987.

Goering, P., Wasylenki, D., Farkas, M., Lancee, W., and Ballantyne, R.: What difference does case management make? *Hospital and Community Psychiatry, 39*(3):272–276, 1988.

Gottlieb, G., and Bloom B.: *Utilization of Specialty Services By Indigent Elderly in Philadelphia.* Philadelphia, Report submitted to the Office of Mental Health and Mental Retardation, 1987.

Hadley, T.R., McGurrin, M.C., Pulice, R., & Holohean, R.: Using fiscal data to identify heavy users. *Psychiatric Quarterly, 61*(1), 41–48, 1990.

Hadley, T.R., McGurrin, M.C., Schinnar, A.P., and Rothbard, A.B. *The Heavy User.* Philadelphia, Report from University of Pennsylvania, Department of Psychiatry, Section on Public Psychiatry & Mental Health Services Research. February, 1988.

Hadley, T.R., Schinnar, A.P., Rothbard, A.B., and Kinosian, M.S.: Capitation financing of public mental health services for the chronically mentally ill. *Administration and Policy in Mental Health, 16*(4):201–214, 1989.

Lehman, A.F.: Capitation payment and mental health care: A review of the opportunities and risks. *Hospital and Community Psychiatry, 38*(1):31–38, 1987.

Lutterman, T.C. Mazade, N.A., Wurster, C.R., and Glover, RW.: Expenditures and revenues of state mental health agencies, 1981–1985. *Hospital and Community Psychiatry, 39:*758–762, 1988.

Mandersheid, R.W., and Barrett, C.A. (Eds.): *Mental Health, U.S., 1987.* Washington, D.C., U.S. Government Printing Office (DHHS Publication No. ADM 87-1518), 1987.

Mauch, D.: Rhode Island: An early effort at managed care. In Mechanic, D. and Aiken, L. (Eds.): *Paying for Services: Promises and Pitfalls of Capitation* (New Directions for Mental health Services Series) San Francisco, Jossey-Bass, 1989, vol. 43, pp. 55–64.

Mechanic, D., and Aiken, L.: Capitation in mental health: Potentials and cautions. In Mechanic, D. and Aiken, L. (Eds.): *Paying for Services: Promises and Pitfalls of Capitation* (New Directions for Mental Health Services Series) San Francisco, Jossey-Bass, 1989, vol. 43, pp. 1–18.

Mechanic, D., and Aiken, L.: Improving the care of patients with chronic mental illness. *The New England Journal of Medicine, 317*(26):1634–1638, 1987.

Morrissey, J.P., and Goldman, H.H.: Cycles of reform in the care of the chronically mentally ill. *Hospital and Community Psychiatry, 35:*785–793, 1984.

Rothbard, A.B., Hadley, T.R., Schinnar, A.P., Morgan, D., and Whitehill, B.: The Philadelphia capitation plan for mental health services. *Hospital and Community Psychiatry, 40:*356–358, 1989.

Schinnar, A.P., and Rothbard, A.B.: Evaluation questions for Philadelphia's mental health capitation experiment. *Hospital and Community Psychiatry, 40:*681–683, 1989.

Schinnar, A.P., Hadley, T.R., and Rothbard, A.B.: *Prediction of Hospitalization in the Philadelphia Mental Health System.* Philadelphia, Report to the Pew Charitable Trust, March, 1988.

Schinnar, A.P., Rothbard, A.B., and Hadley, T.R.: Opportunities and risks in Philadelphia's capitation financing of public funded psychiatric services. *Community Mental Health Journal, 25:*255–266, 1989.

Schlesinger, M.: Striking a balance: Capitation, the mentally ill, and public policy. In Mechanic, D. and Aiken, L. (Eds.): *Paying for Services: Promises and Pitfalls of Capitation* (New Directions for Mental health Services Series) San Francisco, Jossey-Bass, 1989, vol. 43, pp. 97–116.

Schlesinger, M.: On the limits of expanding health care reform: Chronic care in prepaid settings. *Millbank Quarterly, 645*(2):189–215, 1986.

Sharfstein, S.: Medicaid cutbacks and block grants: Crisis or opportunity for community mental health? *American Journal of Psychiatry, 139:*466–470, 1982.

South Carolina Department of Mental Health. *Community Support Demonstration Grant Application,* 1987.

Surles, R.C., and Blanch, A.K.: *Case Management as a Strategy for Systems Change.* Philadelphia, Presented at Innovation and Management in Public Mental Health Systems Conference, Nov. 14, 1989.

Surles, R.C., and McGurrin, M.C.: Increased use of psychiatric emergency services by young chronic mentally ill patients. *Hospital and Community Psychiatry, 38*(4):401–405, 1987.

Talbott, J.A.: The fate of the public psychiatric system. *Hospital and Community Psychiatry, 36*(1):46–50, 1985.

Talbott, J.A., and Sharfstein, S.: A proposal for future funding of chronic and episodic mental illness. *Hospital and Community Psychiatry, 37*(11):1126–1130, 1986.

Thompson, J.W., Bass, R.D., and Witkin, M.J.: Fifty years of psychiatric services: 1940–1990. *Hospital and Community Psychiatry, 33:*711–717, 1986.

Turner, J.C., and Tenhoor, W.J.: The NIMH community support program: Pilot approach to a needed social reform. *Schizophrenia Bulletin, 4:*319–348, 1978.

Worley, N.: Preliminary Report on "Impact of Intensive Case Management on Outcomes for Chronica Mental Illness." NIMH Grant, University of Pennsylvania, School of Nursing, 1989.

Chapter 4

MANAGED MENTAL HEALTH IN HEALTH MAINTENANCE ORGANIZATIONS

Michael J. Bennett

As we enter the final decade of the 20th century, American health care finds itself in disarray. Costs are out of control. Thirty-seven million members of our population have no health insurance. Statistics indicate that we lag behind other western nations in the overall quality, accessibility, and organization of services. The optimism of the 1960s, with its monetary largesse, has given way to the anxious pessimism of the 1990s; the fantasy that free market forces might constrain cost increases while maintaining or enhancing quality has been muted by the harsh realities of the time. Within the mental health field, where cycles of optimism and despair occur with almost predictable regularity (Mechanic, 1987), powerful trends in the diagnosis and treatment of mental disorders muddy the waters even further. Industry clamors for reform, while government vacillates, too burdened by debt and by the legacies of the Reagan years to take any clear initiative in restructuring the health care system.[1]

At the micro level, the privatization of the health care industry has spawned a dazzling multiplicity of health care products, varying in quality and in cost. Physician control, for many years a given, has been replaced by increasing dominance of consumers, employers, and investors as well as regulators. Under scrutiny, health care professionals struggle to redefine their relationships to their patients and clients, and to the payers who represent them. Managed care may be seen as the articulation in practice of the various forces and trends characterized above: an attempt to control and monitor the structure and process of health care in order to influence its outcome, both in regard to quality and cost. One configuration for doing this is the health maintenance organization (HMO).

---

1. The early portion of this chapter is drawn, with permission, from an article that appeared in the *American Journal of Psychiatry*, volume 145: 12, 1988.

In the remainder of this chapter, I will characterize the birth and evolution of the HMO concept and movement, describe the growing variation in structure and mission, and trace the development of mental health programs in HMOs. In considering current trends, I will attempt to place the HMO in its historical context, and suggest how its successes and failures may instruct us in our efforts to create a rational, effective, and affordable mental health component of the health care system.

History of the HMO Movement

As the use of the term "movement" suggests, HMOs originated as reform. Their roots lie in the democratic intent to bring health care to populations of people at affordable cost (Nelson, 1987). The two components, prepayment and group practice have different origins. Prepayment, the provision of a package of services for a prearranged and periodically renegotiated price, began in the early 1900s in the Pacific Northwest, where the lumbering, mining and transportation industries sought to compensate for the unavailability of suitable health care for their employees in the geographically remote areas in which they operated, by hiring their own physicians and treating employees on site. Physicians were salaried, a practice that dates back to the contract physicians of Revolutionary War days. These patterns of care evolved against considerable opposition from organized medicine, eventuating in the "corporate paternalism" (Starr, 1982) associated with companies that sought to maintain the commitment and loyalties of employees through the provision of an array of health and social services. Although the Depression curtailed such programs, they may be seen as forerunners of current trends toward self-insurance and employee assistance programs.

Group practice is generally viewed as originating with the Mayo brothers in the late 1880s. It was not until 1929 that group practice and prepayment were combined. In that year, Ross and Loos contracted with employees of the Los Angeles County Department of Water and Power and their families, offering to provide comprehensive health care services in return for prepaid fees. Their clinic, which expanded to include other industrial groups, is still in operation. At the same time, in rural Oklahoma, a similar venture was initiated by Michael Shadid, a Syrian immigrant with an interest in the relationship between health status and poverty; Shadid negotiated to provide medical care to farmers engaged in cooperatives. In both cases, consumer control was an important feature of the health care partnership. Over the next 40 years, the concept of collaboration and partnership was inherent in the expansion of prepaid group practice. The driving forces behind the organizations later to be known as "first generation HMOs" were industry (Kaiser), consumers (Group Health Cooperative of Puget Sound, Group Health Association of Washington, D.C.), and city government (Health Insurance Plan of Greater New York). With the growth of unionism, organized labor (the Teamsters in St. Louis, United Mine Workers in Appalachia, United Auto Workers in Detroit) became actively involved. Start-up funds were usually drawn from a combination of labor and philanthropic organizations, reflecting the idealism, social purpose and collaborative spirit of the reform movement to that point (Public Health Service, 1974; Mayer and Mayer, 1985). Through the efforts of Walter Reuther, the Community Health Association of Detroit pioneered, in the 1950s, the first development of prepaid mental health services.

The Entry of Government

The Second World War fostered the involvement of government in health care, but it was not until the advent of Medicare and Medicaid in 1965 that government became a direct payer. Through the 1960s, with its emphasis on human rights, its idealism, its "Great Society," health care initiatives and costs burgeoned (Starr, 1982). In its quest for cost containment, the Nixon administration engaged Paul Ellwood who articulated the strategy that was to become the centerpiece of the Nixon health care policy. Ellwood, who was at that time the executive director of the American Rehabilitation Institute, argued that the fee-for-service system provided no incentive for preventive and rehabilitative care, since physicians were rewarded only for treating illness. By contrast, prepaid group practices such as Kaiser, which he dubbed "health maintenance organizations" (Mayer and Mayer, 1985), were strongly motivated, by the nature of their financial imperatives, to keep their members from becoming or remaining ill. Observing the financial success of Kaiser, with no apparent sacrifice in quality, Ellwood advocated that the government abandon the heretofore unsuccessful policy of central control in favor of investing in a network of comprehensive prepaid group practices. This strategy, designed to transform the health care system and promote cost containment, was inherently competitive. The pro-competitive strategy was more fully articulated later, by Enthoven: health care costs could be contained best in a free-market system, which de-emphasized regulation by relying on a multiplicity of health care entities of varying nature to compete with each other for consumers, whose buying choices would act as a brake on escalating costs (Starr, 1982).

These ideas were adopted by the Nixon administration, leading to the HMO Act of 1973 (PL 93-222). This act subsidized the creation and expansion of HMOs, but modified their nature in two ways: First, profit-making corporations, not significantly associated with the HMO movement to that point, were welcomed. Second, the door was opened to the "medical care foundation," forerunner of the independent practice association (IPA). This structure originated in 1954 with the San Joaquin Foundation for Medical Care, an affiliation of physicians in office prac- tice who agreed to fixed fees without creating a formal group structure (Mayer and Mayer, 1985). Modern IPAs are considered one of the three classical varieties of HMO. They preserve the structure of fee-for-service medicine while introducing prepayment. By contrast, the other two classical structures, group and staff model HMOs, preponderant to that point, consist of health care providers who are linked to each other as well as to the organization that supplies enrollees as patients. This linkage may take the form of shared employment (staff model) or formal partnership or corporate status (group model, or its extension, a network: a group of such groups). These structural differences exert a profound influence on participating providers and affect their practice in various ways, to be described later.

As a consequence of government's use and reshaping of the HMO movement, its fundamental nature was irretrievably altered. As Starr (1982) has commented, "A remarkable change had taken place. Prepaid group practice was originally associated with the cooperative movement and dismissed as a utopian, slightly subversive idea. The conservative, cost-minded critics of medical care had now adopted it as a more effi- cient form of management. They had substituted a rhetoric of rationaliza- tion and competition for the older rhetoric of cooperation and mutual protection. The socialized medicine of one era had become the corporate reform of the next".

Mental Health Care in HMOs

Prepaid mental health care is a relatively new phenomenon. Despite their commitment to comprehensive care, the early HMOs, with the exception of the St. Louis Labor Institute, remained wary of mental health care or coverage. The Health Insurance Plan of Greater New York provided only diagnosis and consultation, while Kaiser arranged for fee-for-service care for its members on a reduced fee basis. Such wariness was also characteristic of the indemnity insurance sector. It was based on a distrust of mental health diagnosis and treatment and a fear of the "bottomless pit" of costs that might be incurred with less restrictive policies.

In response to such concerns, a number of studies were carried out in the 1960s, beginning with Helen Avnet, demonstrating the affordability of a limited mental health benefit (Avnet, 1962). The first inclusion of mental health benefits on an optional or rider basis began in response to the influence of large contractor groups: the Federal Employees Health Benefits Program, Medicare, Medicaid, and union and employee groups. By the late 1960s, second generation plans (Harvard Community Health Plan, the Community Health Care Center Plan of New Haven, and the Columbia Medical Plan) decided to include substantial mental health care as a basic benefit. Later, with passage of the HMO Act, and in order to benefit from the advantages of federal qualification, other plans were forced to include basic mental health benefits as well. Reflecting the HMO industry's ambivalent and therefore unenthusiastic support, the HMO Act required only minimal benefits. These included crisis intervention and evaluative services (up to 20 visits), not inpatient care, and not benefits for chronic or recurrent conditions or for chemical dependency. It is important to note that many plans found such exclusions unnecessary or unworkable, and a number developed broader benefit packages. Most commonly, inpatient benefits were for 30 days per year, with partial inpatient care expanding coverage to 60. Sixteen years later, such packages remain the norm.

Since most early programs developed in staff or group model structures, which are closed systems, cost containment mechanisms were intrinsic. Certain strategies, such as the substitution of lower for higher cost personnel and the control of staff-to-patient ratios were common. Mental health program costs were also contained through barriers to access (copayments, gatekeeper functions assigned to medical or primary care providers, exclusions of the chronically ill in some cases), or through offering treatment programs suitable for only some of the membership (for example, no programs for the chemically dependent). These structural features tended to shape provider function. For example, settings such as the Community Health Care Center Program, which emphasized a strong primary care mental health role, developed active teaching and liaison initiatives to facilitate such a function on the part of internists and pediatricians (Bennett and Gavalya, 1982; Coleman, Patrick and Baker, 1977). The structure and organization of mental health services varied from highly integrated models (Harvard Community Health Plan) to off-site, centralized programs (Health Insurance Plan of Greater New York). In some instances, services were contracted out—for example, to community mental health centers. Benefits and services gradually expanded, in response to consumer and staff demand, increasing acceptance in the community, and demonstrated ability to manage costs. A number of states enacted legislation requiring a broadening of benefits and services beyond the federal requirement.

Through the 1970s and early 1980s, the closed panel HMO became a distinctive form of mental health practice, characterized by similar values, practice patterns, and programs, i.e., a common culture (Budman, Feldman and Bennett, 1979; Bittker and Idzorek, 1978; Spoerl, 1974). Certain elements of context favored this. First, members and staff both tended to select the HMO knowingly, attracted to it for specific reasons. In the case of staff, there was often a spirit of idealism, innovation, and career risk involvement. Professionals working in HMOs were regarded by peers in the community with suspicion and skepticism. Attracted by the opportunity for single class, population-based care, or the chance to be innovative, they were forced to reconcile their training with the constraints and opportunities of the setting, and to find new ways of operating. Second, members joined HMOs voluntarily, often with some awareness of the advantages and disadvantages involved. This favored alliance with staff seeking to be innovative rather than traditional. Programs shared certain characteristics: (1) rediscovery of the effectiveness of brief and intermittent types of psychotherapy, which were considered suitable not only for selected patients, but for a diverse population; (2) emphasis on timely and ready access to necessary services, (3) use, where clinically possible, of outpatient or partial outpatient care rather than full inpatient care; (4) renewed interest in liaison psychiatry in the outpatient general medical setting as a way of enhancing the general medical provider's role in mental health care; (5) emphasis on collaborative rather than solo practice; and (6) eclecticism, i.e., the use or adaptation of a variety of treatment methods compatible with cost effectiveness. Among other things, this spawned a renewed interest in group, including brief group, therapy.

The Present Environment

With the continued success of the HMO movement, fundamental changes began to occur. By 1987, there were over 600 plans with close to 30 million enrollees. It has been predicted that by the year 1993, 50 million Americans will be members of HMOs, and experts predict that in the 1990s, the majority of the U.S. population will be enrolled in some form of price-competitive plan (Flinn, McMahon, and Collins, 1987). Along with rapid growth, there has been a loss of the purity of design, and multiple variations in structure now exist. In addition, as HMOs have become mainstream, changes in public expectations have led to alterations in organizational identity and mission. These changes have been accelerated by the increasing importance of capital in the health care industry, and by the changes in ownership of that capital. With the pro-competitive scenario in full bloom, a multiplicity of players have entered the health care marketplace and health care has become "monetarized" (Ginzberg, 1984); increasingly dominated by those whose primary business is business, the accumulation and preservation of capital. If yesterday's HMO was designed to organize and deliver health care, today's is likely to be a "product line," one activity of an organization seeking to survive and prosper in the marketplace. These alterations have profoundly affected the nature of practice in general, and mental health practice in particular.

Changing Structure

Currently there is a trend toward open systems. In 1984–85, 71% of the 92 new HMOs were IPAs (Flinn, McMahon and Collins, 1987), which account for over 60% of all HMOs and over 40% of all HMO enrollees (Page, 1987). This trend appears to be continuing. In addition, preferred provider organizations (PPOs), in which a provider group offers a discount for insured services, with the insured having the choice of paying standard fees by selecting a provider who is not a member of the PPO, are becoming affiliated with HMOs (or evolving into them). In both the PPO and IPA structure, with only the latter being prepaid, professionals practice geographically remote from each other (and from the insurer), usually in their own offices. The closed panel system, by telescoping the three components of health care, the consumer, the provider and the insurer, creates an opportunity for a give and take among them and for the establishment of a culture that is shaped by their overlapping interests.

By contrast, open systems accentuate the often competing agendas of these three interest groups, and call for external mechanisms to link them.

There are several important implications for mental health care. As one of the fastest growing cost components of health care, mental health remains a special concern of the purchaser (primarily those who represent the consumer). In some instances, this has led industry to carve out mental health and chemical dependency programs and to separate them from general health care (Martinsons, 1988), reflecting disenchantment with benefits and services, and especially with the failure to contain cost. Cost is closely linked to the ability to control utilization. Lacking internal mechanisms to do so, open systems must rely on benefit constraints, cost-sharing, and checks on provider behavior. These are often retrospective and can be intrusive or even adversarial. One emerging answer to the cost containment problem is for the organization to subcontract the management function to a managed care company that specializes in monitoring patient and provider behavior. Financial arrangements usually involve some form of risk sharing. In still another variation, many HMOs wishing to divest themselves of the risk involved in mental health care choose to subcontract the delivery function as well, to selected hospitals, community mental health centers, or preferred vendor groups. In contrast to the relatively uniform cultures of the closed systems of the 1970s, such arrangements are likely to emphasize control rather than education, alliance and collaboration.

For providers engaged in an open system, who may be poorly prepared by standard training for the demands and constraints of prepaid practice, or who may be involved primarily for economic reasons, and who therefore are likely to view other providers as competitors rather than as collaborators, efficient practice patterns may prove difficult to achieve. First, lacking the supports and the incentive to be innovative, they are likely to use abbreviated traditional methods instead, relying heavily on time-intensive (psychodynamic, usually individual) forms of psychotherapy. As the clinical literature suggests (Bennett, 1989; Budman and Gurman, 1988), there is a considerable difference between planned brevity and simply limiting the number of sessions of psychotherapy. Moreover, the individual provider who is compensated on a per visit basis may have little incentive to refer to colleagues for specialized focal methodology, relying instead on methods with which he or she is familiar, whether or not these are the most expeditious for the given clinical situation. One survey of 145 HMOs nationally revealed a strong link between structure and services programs, with IPAs offering fewer and more traditional services than staff or group models (Cheifetz and Solloway, 1984). Since it appears that managerial attitudes and policies may be the most crucial determinants of access, use and utilization of mental health services (rather than benefits, per se) (Brady and Krizay, 1985), the distancing of management from practice, and therefore from the give and take of face-to-face contact, carries the risk of underemphasizing provider and consumer agendas in favor of narrowly defined managerial interests. (Many staff model HMOs seek to avoid such narrowing of perspective by insisting that physician managers continue to practice.) It is widely hoped that the development of quality assessment technology will create protection against such risks, but such technology is not sufficiently developed or available at the present time to be used in this way.

Changing Expectations

The change in expectations has two root causes. First, the HMO has been seized upon not only as a viable option for a segment of the population that is oriented toward its advantages and willing to accept its limitations, but as a panacea for the health care needs of the population at large. As the history of expectation and disappointment in the community health center movement indicates (Donovan, 1982), good ideas can be oversold. Second, in a competitive environment characterized by slick advertising and fierce competition, limitations are de-emphasized.

The activities of HMOs have become a focus of national attention. No longer the "new kid on the block," and no longer viewed even by their adherents as capable of stemming the inflationary tide, HMOs are forced to justify their cost/service and cost/quality trade-offs to regulators, increasingly powerful consumer interest groups, and to industrial purchasers. As health care providers to a large and growing segment of the population, HMOs are expected to offer appropriate and adequate services to the costly and difficult to manage clinical challenges of our age: AIDS, chemical dependence, problems of aging, major and chronic mental illness. These growing priorities threaten programs traditionally associated with HMO practice: primary ambulatory services, well-child (and to some extent, well-adult) services, secondary and tertiary prevention. With dramatic shifts in fee-for-service patterns, the traditional gap between prepaid and fee-for-service systems in regard to inpatient costs has been much reduced, forcing HMOs to become more efficient in order to compete with the fee-for-service and indemnity sector and with each other.

With regard to mental health, current pressures to enroll the chronically mentally ill have been spurred in part by the promises of prepayment and the success of closed panel organizations in containing costs in the past, and in part by the concurrent underfunding and desiccation of the public sector. As Schlesinger (1986) has pointed out, however, the three perceived advantages of prepaid systems—reduction of hospital days, better coordination of care, and prevention—will not automatically occur in the absence of specific planning and funding. These are usually lacking. A variety of proposals have been made, some quite creative (Lehman, 1987), but most HMOs that offer services to the chronically ill (and most HMOs continue to exclude this part of the population), are likely to have to squeeze such patients into the available medical framework, one that underemphasizes their crucial human service needs. Further, with the emphasis on member initiative, and the relatively passive approach of most HMOs to health education and outreach, it is unlikely that this population will come to attention early enough and readily enough to be well served. Funneling money into the private sector for such purposes is likely to exacerbate the problem of underfunding in the public sector. The prospect of cooperation between the two is unlikely at present, given the uneasy relationship that exists between them in most parts of the country.

Changing Mission: Monetarization or 'Greening' Of The HMO

It is not unusual, in our culture, for reform movements to be "discovered" and exploited for their economic potential. Writing about the feminist movement in the Boston Globe, Suzanne Gordon (1988) states, "Unfortunately, almost as soon as feminism began to make some progress its edge was dulled. What happened, not surprisingly in a consumer-oriented society, was that mainstream America quickly turned a powerful social movement into a vast and lucrative new market."

Health care, similarly, has become a commodity rather than an end-in-itself (Levey and Hesse, 1985). This is suggested by the reconfiguration of delivery systems to find niches in the marketplace, the emphasis on competition to determine pricing for goods and services, and the growth of investor-owned systems. Profitability has become the yardstick of performance and health centers have evolved into profit centers (Starr, 1982). HMO development, classically characterized by high initial investment, long start-up times, and slow growth, now is likely to occur by merger or acquisition. HMOs originate and disappear, introducing volatility into an activity requiring consistency and predictability. Benefit variations, options, and the mix of fee-for-service and prepaid patients characteristic of most IPA practice create a confusing array of possibilities for the patient and provider that must be factored into clinical planning. These factors have introduced three overlapping elements into HMO practice: First, an emphasis on the competitive ethic and on profit; second, the professionalization of health care management; and third, a preoccupation with the quantitative and technical (measurable) dimensions of practice, at the cost of those dimensions that are less so. All three have implications for mental health practice.

The practice of medicine is a collaborative enterprise. This is best articulated in the psychotherapeutic concept of therapeutic alliance. Organizational policies too strongly attuned to the "bottom line" threaten the necessary subjugation of self-interest and acquisitiveness and place the provider in a potential conflict-of-interest situation. Decisions to fund or to withhold funding of programs or to care for or withhold care from subsets of the population based on profitability strike at the heart of medical ethics. When pressure to undersell the competition leads to underpricing, undertreatment may be the result. As Starr (1982) has commented, professionalism requires a behavioral code that exceeds marketplace ethics; efforts to standardize practice and eliminate waste and inefficiency are laudable, while efforts at corporate socialization of providers carries the risk of undermining professionalism in favor of marketplace standards.

Success in today's health care arena requires sound business practice. In order to insure this, HMOs have invested greatly in the development of a cadre of managers, including medical managers, who are well versed in business principles. In that sense, managerial function has been professionalized. Providers who are employees surrender a part of their customary autonomy and, in closed systems, operate under the surveillance of on-site managers whose expectations for productivity, efficiency, and fulfillment of job performance standards mirror similar management-employee dynamics in non-health care industry. In open systems, managerial functions may be exercised less directly, with emphasis on measurable parameters of function; this exaggerates the value of quantifiable dimensions of practice (numbers of patients seen, numbers of new patients accommodated, hours filled, etc.) with implicit de-emphasis of the qualitative aspects of practice (Bennett, 1988a).

These matters are of great relevance to mental health professionals, whose work frequently involves activities (such as psychotherapy) that may be difficult or impossible to monitor with purely quantitative measures. Shaped by such forces, mental health programs are likely to emphasize time-efficient approaches even more strongly: biological and symptom-alleviating methodology at the expense of the psychosocial dimension of practice, even dynamic forms of brief psychotherapy.

It is largely these pressures that have forced many health care providers to ally with each other, to take the initiative in forming PPOs and IPAs, and to resist or carefully negotiate contractual relationships with HMOs, fearing too great a loss of autonomy and too great a need to reshape professional values. Ironically, even such protective responses have contributed to the trends that are reshaping practice.

Current Patterns of Mental Health Care

It is a persistent complaint of those not associated with HMOs that they achieve their success through favorable selection. There is no convincing evidence for this. In addition, critics claim that HMOs limit their benefits, erect barriers to necessary care (and thus undertreat), and that they sacrifice quality for cost considerations. A number of surveys and studies have appeared in the literature over the last several years, attempting to assess such claims. The Rand Study compared the patterns of care at Group Health Cooperative of Puget Sound, a large closed panel HMO, with fee-for-service practice given similar benefits and costs. As with other studies of the last 30 years, they found no difference in measurable quality but found costs lower in the HMO. Luft has commented that this study, as well as earlier ones, may be deceptive in that it uses an older, closed panel HMO which may no longer be typical (1988). In regard to psychotherapy, the Rand study found differences in intensity; that is, fee-for-service patients were as likely as prepaid patients to seek help from a mental health professional, but the fee-for-service patients used more service (and thus incurred higher costs) (Wells, Manning and Benjamin, 1986a, 1987). Since Group Health emphasizes family practice, with a prominent role for medical providers in mental health care, prepaid members had a greater likelihood of receiving some form of care for their problems, being more likely than their fee-for-service counterparts to use a non-mental health provider, while using mental health professionals at about the same rate. It is not clear how the mental health care received from medical providers compares in nature or effectiveness with that provided by mental health specialists. Costs were considerably less in the HMO population, because of greater use of non-physician mental health personnel, more use of group and other lower cost methodology and fewer visits per patient. The same study demonstrated that children were somewhat more likely to receive service in the HMO (Wells, Manning and Benjamin, 1986b), and that poor people with significant health problems did better in the fee-for-service system, while the non-poor and the poor who were healthy did about the same. It was speculated that the difference for the sick poor was in the lack of outreach in the HMO (Ware, Brook, Rogers, Keeler, Davies, Sherbourne, Goldberg and Camp, 1986), a finding with considerable significance in regard to enrolling the chronically mentally ill in pre-paid systems.

The Rand Study also indicated that HMO enrollees were as likely to visit a mental health specialist in a given year, but 50% more likely to do so over several years; fee-for-service patients, by contrast, remained in treatment longer (Manning, Wells and Benjamin, 1987). These findings are consistent with typical HMO patterns of care, in that focal or brief treatment is likely to be employed by design, and patients may and do return. There is a growing clinical literature, which comes mainly from HMOs, that describes this pattern (Bennett, 1983; Siddall, Haffey and Feinman, 1988).

Levin has conducted three national surveys of HMO coverage and utilization, in 1978, 1982, and 1986 (Levin, Glasser and Roberts, 1984, 1988). He has found trends toward greater inclusion of mental health services and services for substance abuse, with his latest survey indicating 97% of respondents offering mental health coverage and two thirds, alcohol and substance abuse benefits or services. In all three studies, Levin confirmed that early wariness (as reflected in the cautious, limited mental health benefit requirement of the federal HMO Act of 1973) had persisted. The most common package remains the standard 20 outpatient and 30 day inpatient benefit. Interestingly, Levin found that outpatient costs had remained the same while inpatient costs had risen considerably over the years, as a product of more inpatient days. In contrast to the

1982 study, which found a mean hospital utilization figure of 32 days per thousand members per year and mean ambulatory utilization of .33 encounters per member per year, the 1986 study found figures of 36 days per thousand members per year and .22 encounters. It is likely that this reflects a change in the covered population, which is probably considerably less favorably selected than in earlier years, and perhaps some loss of initiative in designing outpatient alternatives to inpatient care. Since chemical dependency costs are often subsumed under mental health care, it may also reflect the exacerbation of problems and greater investment in treatment for this population.

A number of authors have commented on the HMO practice of limiting mental health benefits and continuing to make a distinction between mental health and general medical coverage. It is interesting to note that many states, in response to growing concerns about the adequacy of benefits, have enacted legislation mandating minimal benefits. Levin studied mental health and substance abuse patterns in HMOs in the 40 states which have mandated minimal benefits. He found that 27 of these regulated mental health benefits, 38 did so for alcohol and drug abuse; 22 of those regulating mental health benefits did so specifically for HMOs, indicating concern. In addition, states without mandatory legislation regulated HMO mental health benefits despite the absence of general legislation (Levin, 1988). It is not clear how effective such legislation is; as Seltzer (1988) has noted, such minimal benefits are likely to become the ceiling rather than the floor.

Although no similar current information is available on staffing patterns, there is evidence that HMOs use non physician personnel extensively. Psychologists, who function as psychotherapists, are also likely to be involved in research programs when they exist, and it is suggested that they may also be more involved in educational and behavioral medicine initiatives than their mental health colleagues (DeLeon, Uyeda and Welch, 1985; Tulkin and Frank, 1985). Especially in closed panel settings, where the use of interdisciplinary teams has been one method used traditionally to contain costs, social workers, psychiatric nurses and substance abuse specialists play prominent roles. Interdisciplinary function is probably a good deal less common in IPAs and PPOs, where the composition of the provider group is more likely to be homogeneous. This may account for the reduced range of treatment options in IPAs (Cheifetz and Solloway, 1984), since the different mental health disciplines are likely to emphasize expertise in different, though overlapping, strategies of treatment. A richer mix of treatment philosophies and strategies is likely to produce a more eclectic and varied mental health program.

In contrast to the 8% of the cost for all medical care that is spent on mental health (the amount appears to be increasing, particularly for large employers) in the fee-for-service sector, the common figure in HMOs is 3 to 5% (Martinsons, 1985). Given the rise in costs discovered by Levin, the trend may be upward. As open systems become a larger share of the HMO market, with their greater difficulty in integrating the levels of care and in coordinating care at any given level, these figures may increase further. To some extent, this will depend on how well evolving techniques for managing health care in such systems prove able to control provider and patient behavior and contain burgeoning costs. A growing awareness on the part of medical schools and other training institutions of the economics of health care, greater pressure on students to learn and providers to practice cost-effective patterns of care, and further shifts in the dominant pattern of mental health practice from time-intensive to population-based and cost-effective methods may counteract this somewhat. Marshall (1987), in a thoughtful and optimistic review of the impact of HMOs on general psychiatric practice, concludes that there may be a "silver lining." He observes that the conditions of prepaid practice incline us toward a narrower definition of what constitutes mental disorder, and greater flexibility in the use of methodology, with less tendency to persist in patterns of treatment that are not working. He predicts that the psychotherapies will become less exotic and more problem oriented, with greater standardization and with a shift from continuous, long-term forms of therapy to intermittent models of care. This is consistent with a series of articles from the HMO community, describing such patterns of care, referred to above.

Implications For The Future

With growing pressure on employers to provide health insurance and on the general taxpayer to solve the problem of the uninsured, and with the continuing escalation of general health and mental health costs, a crisis appears imminent. Legislators, employers, consumers, and public sector officials, whose interests overlap, will be forced to reshape the system in ways that may sharply differ from both the current pro-competitive scenario and from the circumstances preceding it. One example is recent legislation enacted in the state of Oregon, rationing health care services to the indigent. This law establishes a commission composed of consumers, physicians and other health care practitioners (including a minority of M.D.s) that has the task of prioritizing health care options for an expanding pool of welfare recipients, so that a limited budget may be allocated in a consistent and pre-determined manner. One requirement of this legislation is that the health care be provided primarily by managed care systems. Although the Oregon law will not affect mental health or chemical dependency services, it is a bold step that is sure to be watched carefully by health planners everywhere. Similar initiatives are underway in other areas (Lund, 1989). The move to diagnosis-related groups (DRGs), like capitation, rationalizes health care expenditures by linking treatment options to allocated costs, and therefore places greater emphasis on cost projection at the systems level and treatment planning at the individual patient level. Such initiatives lay the groundwork for necessary reforms in the pricing of mental health services, and for rethinking the matter of affordability of adequate mental health care for the population at large.

The coming era will be characterized by a better informed consumer, whose leverage over the health care system will be exercised by purchase decisions, made either by the consumer or by those who represent his or her interest (Sharfstein, Krizay, and Muszynski, 1988). HMOs, if they are to survive and prosper, will have to adapt to the changing environment. The confusing multiplicity of options available in the health care marketplace reflects this effort to adapt. Today's consumer may elect a variety of insurance options within the same organization, either choosing in advance or at the point of service, weighing the importance of choice of provider or treatment method versus cost of service. For the most part, the public and the private sector remain sharply separate, each responding to the competitive pressures by increasing scrutiny of services and frequently by curtailing them. Progressive cutbacks in public funding and the growing pressure to move patients from the public into the private sector will eventually bring this situation to a head. HMOs that have negotiated capitation arrangements with public facilities may be one harbinger of necessary change.

Carve-outs, the growing practice of separating one component of health care from others, usually involve a fourth party, a company that contracts to manage that element of care; frequently it is mental health care. Because such management companies must develop mechanisms for shaping provider behavior to bring it more in line with cost objectives, some are turning more to education of providers in an effort to induce practice patterns that are reminiscent of the cultures of staff model HMOs; in some instances, existing groups of providers are involved, while in others, such groups may be newly created (Herrington, 1989). As with any open system, integration of the treatment alternatives at a given level of care (horizontal integration) or at the interfaces between levels of care (vertical integration) can be a major problem.

The ability to separate mental health from other health care may have advantages if the capitation is fair and reasonable. Specialized resources and facilities for mental health may be developed without the need to compete with other agendas of the general medical setting; in addition, a better general understanding of the requirements for good mental health care may be possible, with appropriate emphasis on its non-medical dimensions. Along with this, better attention may be paid to the interface with other mental health resources in the surrounding community. In contrast to the IPA, and similar to the closed panel HMO, managed mental health care that is provided apart from the general medical setting is likely to involve a mix of professionals whose activities are linked to each other in cost conserving ways.

The risk of such "carve-outs" is the return to fragmented care, with mental health once again seen as distinct from general medical care, impoverishing both. Opportunities for teaching medical providers to practice sound mental health care within their medical practices may be reduced, if not lost. Finally, the reservoir of patients will be limited to those who choose to define themselves as mentally ill, interposing a barrier to necessary mental health care for the large number of patients who bring their emotional disorders to the medical provider and may resist referral. Of course, bridges can be built to general health care providers and services, but the prepayment mechanism does not encourage case finding. Without greater prioritization of prevention, health education, and early intervention that current funding mechanisms encourage, the trend toward carving out mental health services is hazardous. One hopeful element is the relationship that often exists between employers and mental health management companies. In some instances, this is manifest in linkages between in-house (for example, employee assistance programs) and out-of-house programs and providers. Such linkages offer the possibility of better case finding and aftercare options, and better leverage in gaining employee collaboration with the goals of mental health care.

Given the current national mood, characterized by preoccupation with the national debt combined with resistance to raising general taxes, the trend of callous and self-defeating curtailment of human service programs at the national and state level is likely to continue in the immediate future. At the level of health care policymaking, this will be reflected in further constriction of funding for the human service elements in health care. Balancing this, however, there is growing awareness of the costs associated with untreated mental and chemical dependency disorders, and considerable pressure on the part of industry to prioritize such treatment. Once again, funding is likely to favor existing and evolving biological techniques, leading to an even greater tendency to "medicalize" mental health and chemical dependency care.

In addition to such "medicalization," three other trends are likely to be of considerable importance in shaping tomorrow's mental health programs: greater emphasis on population-based care; increasing use of computer and other technology to improve the efficiency and ergonomics of care; and an increasing emphasis on educating the consumer and involving him or her in self-care. Population-based care, in which the needs of the individual patient are balanced with responsibility for a broader population (for an HMO, the membership; for society in general, the pool of prospective patients) is the most problematic, in that it involves a fundamental shift away from the dyadic relationship upon which most mental health care in this century has been based. Although population-based care favors case-finding, early intervention and prevention, such strategies are costly to implement and usually not of proven value in the mental health field. In this era of rationing, with pressure to make health care available to larger numbers of people while keeping costs in check, planners are more likely to favor group and self-help approaches and treatment in context: in the home and family, in the workplace, in the community. They, along with health care purchasers, will endorse limited and clear treatment objectives and procedures of proven effectiveness over those that may help some, but cannot be demonstrated to be effective for the population at large. Such changes will call for improved organization and coordination of services, putting better integrated and better managed delivery systems at a competitive advantage. Such factors may mitigate or even reverse the current trend toward open systems; that may be seen as an attempt to preserve the structure of medical care in the face of demands to modify its financing. Ultimately, structure will be forced to change as well.

As an experiment in health care, yesterday's "pure" HMO is gone, replaced by the hybrid organizations of today and the increasingly mixed ones of the future. What have we learned? First, although the issue is far from settled, it does appear that mental health care is insurable: i.e., affordable. Second, that there are tradeoffs (offset) between mental health and general health care services, and that the withholding of necessary mental health care is a foolish economy (Bennett, 1988b) Third, the integration of the mental health disciplines, and the integration of mental health and general health care services offers the potential for comprehensive care, for early (and therefore probably briefer) intervention, and for enlarging the pool of mental health patients to include those who characteristically remain within the general medical setting.

We have also learned that the HMO setting produces problems for mental health care. Forced to compete with the priorities of the general health care setting, and to operate within the value systems and models of care common to the medical setting, mental health often does not fare well. There is a tendency to underfund and to "medicalize": to rely excessively on active interventions and on techniques of diagnosis and treatment that emphasize the biological, sometimes at the expense of the human service elements of care. Chronic patients, often excluded from HMOs, at times by criteria that exaggerate the prognostic significance of formal diagnosis, may not receive adequate care even when included. Their needs are likely to be oversimplified, and it is common for their care to "spill over" into the public sector, not by design or coordination, but by exclusion or exhaustion of limited benefits. Gatekeepers, usually referring medical providers, may act as barriers rather than as conduits, and may offer no effective care to the patient discouraged from seeing a specialist. Unfortunately, the greatest promise of the HMO for mental health care, a true equality with medical illness and care, has never been achieved.

By borrowing what has been learned from the HMO setting and capitalizing on its strengths and achievements, tomorrow's managed care can further advance the caliber, accessibility, and affordability of care. Achieving this requires advances in characterizing and assessing quality in mental health care. If the twin objectives of the HMO movement, affordability and accessibility, are to be realized, all players in the health care drama must be given adequate voice. The conscience of society, as reflected in the behavior of its elected representatives, will have to monitor and limit the profit motif. If an appropriate blend of competition and collaboration can be forged, perhaps some of the idealism associated with the HMO movement, dampened over the years by the realities of cost, chronicity, and limited knowledge, may be rekindled in its successors.

REFERENCES

Avnet, H.H.: *Psychiatric Insurance.* New York, Group Health Insurance, 1962.

Bennett, M.J., and Gavalya, A.: Prepaid comprehensive mental health services for children. *J Am Acad Child Psychiatry, 21:*486–491, 1982.

Bennett, M.J.: Focal psychotherapy: terminable and interminable. *Am J Psychotherapy, 37:*365–375, 1983.

Bennett, M.J.: The greening of the HMO: implications for prepaid psychiatry. *Am J Psychiatry, 145:*1544–1549, 1988a.

Bennett, M.J.: Quality assurance activities for mental health services in health maintenance organizations. In Stricker G. and Rodriguez A. (Eds): *Handbook of Quality Assurance in Mental Health.* New York, Plenum, 1988b.

Bennett, M.J.: The catalytic function in psychotherapy. *Psychiatry, 52:*351–364, 1989.

Bittker, T.E., and Idzorek, S.: The evolution of psychiatric services in a health maintenance organization. *Am J Psychiatry, 135:*339–342, 1978.

Brady, J., and Krizay, J.: Utilization and coverage of mental health services in health maintenance organizations. *Am J Psychiatry, 142:*744–746, 1985.

Budman, S.H., Feldman, J., and Bennett, M.J.: Adult mental health services in a health maintenance organization. *Am J Psychiatry, 136:*392–395, 1979.

Budman, S.H., and Gurman, A.S.: *Theory and Practice of Brief Therapy.* New York, Guilford, 1988, pp 6–9.

Cheifetz, D.I., and Solloway, J.C.: Patterns of mental health services provided by HMOs. *Am Psychol, 39:*495–502, 1984.

Coleman, J., Patrick, D., and Baker, S.: The mental health of children in an HMO program. *Pediatrics, 91:*150–153, 1977.

DeLeon, P.H., Uyeda, M.K., and Welch, B.L.: Psychology and HMOs: new partnership or new adversary? *Am Psychol, 40:*1122–1124, 1985.

Donovan, C.M.: Problems of psychiatric practice in community mental health centers. *Am J Psychiatry, 139:*456–460, 1982.

Flinn, D., McMahon, T., and Collins, M.: Health maintenance organizations and their implications for psychiatry. *Hosp Community Psychiatry, 38:*255–263, 1987.

Ginzberg, E.: The monetarization of medical care. *N Engl J Med, 310:*1162–1165, 1984.

Gordon, S.: Feminism goes to market. *Boston Globe,* October 18, 1988, p. 35.

Herrington, B.S.: "Carving out" mental health: new way to provide care. *Psych News,* July 7, 1989, p9.

Levey, S., and Hesse, D.D.: Bottom-line health care? *N Engl J Med, 312:*644–647, 1985.

Levin, B.L.: State mandates for mental health, alcohol and substance abuse benefits: implications for HMOs. *GHAA Journal, 9:*48–69, 1988.

Levin, B.L., Glasser, J.H., and Roberts, RE: Changing patterns in mental health service coverage within health maintenance organizations. *Am J Public Health, 74:*453–458, 1984.

Levin, B.L., Glasser, J.H., and Roberts, R.E.: National trends in coverage and utilization of mental health, alcohol, and substance abuse services within managed health care systems. *Am J Pub Health, 78:*1222–1223, 1988.

Luft, H.S.: HMOs and the quality of care. *Inquiry, 25:*145–156, 1988.

Lund, D.S.: Health care rationing plan ok'd in Oregon; stymied in California. *Am Med News,* July 21, 1989, p 1.

Manning, W.G., Wells, K.B., and Benjamin, B.: Use of outpatient mental health services over time in a health maintenance organization and fee-for-service plans. *Am J Psychiatry, 144:*283–287, 1987.

Marshall, J.R.: HMOs and psychiatry—could there be a silver lining? *Int J Law Psychiatry, 10:*35–43, 1987.

Martinsons, J.N.: Are HMOs slamming the door on psych treatment? *Hospitals,* March 5, 62:50–56, 1988.

Mayer, T.R., and Mayer, G.G.: HMOs: origins and development. *N Engl J Med, 312:*590–594, 1985.

Mechanic, D. (Ed): Evolution of mental health services and areas for change. In Improving mental health services: what the social sciences can tell us. In *New Directions for Mental Health Services, 36:*3–13, 1987.

Nelson, J.: The history and spirit of the HMO movement. *HMO Practice, 1:*75–85, 1987.

Page, L.: Report notes impact of alternative delivery systems. *Am Med News,* Dec. 18, 1987, p. 12.

Inclusion of Mental Health Services in Health Maintenance Organizations: A Review of Supplemental Benefits, DHEW Publication HSA 75-13019. Washington, DC, U.S. Department of Health, Education and Welfare, Public Health Service, 1974.

Schlesinger, M.: On the limits of expanding health care reform: chronic care in prepaid settings. *Milbank Q, 64:*189–215, 1986.

Seltzer, D.A.: Limitations on HMO services and the emerging redefinition of chronic mental illness. *Hosp Community Psychiatry, 39:*137–139, 1988.

Sharfstein, S.S., Krizay, J., and Muszynski, J.D.: Defining and pricing psychiatric care "products." *Hosp Community Psychiatry, 39:*372–375. 1988.

Siddall, L.B., Haffey, N.A., and Feinman, J.A.: Intermittent brief psychotherapy in an HMO setting. *Am J Psychotherapy, 42:*96–106, 1988.

Spoerl, O.H.: Treatment patterns in prepaid psychiatric care. *Am J Psychiatry, 131:*56–59, 1974.

Starr, P.: *The Social Transformation of American Medicine.* New York, Basic Books, 1982.

Tulkin, S.R., and Frank, G.W.: The changing role of psychologists in health maintenance organizations. *Am Psychol, 4:*1125–1130, 1985.

Ware, J.E., Brook, R.H., Rogers, W.H., Keeler, E.B., Davies, A.R., Sherbourne, C.D., Goldberg, G.A., and Camp, P.: Comparison of health outcomes at a health maintenance organisation with those of fee-for-service care. *Lancet, 1:*1017–1022, 1986.

Wells, K.B., Manning, W.F., and Benjamin, B.: Use of outpatient mental health services in HMO and fee-for-service plans: results from a randomized controlled trial. *Health Serv Res, 21:*453–474, 1986a.

Wells, K.B., Manning, W.F., and Benjamin, B.: A comparison of the effects of sociodemographic factors and health status on use of outpatient mental health services in HMO and fee-for-service plans. *Med Care, 24:*949–960, 1986b

Wells, K.B., Manning, W.F., and Benjamin, B.: A comparison of use of outpatient mental health services in an HMO and fee-for-service plans. *Med Care, 25:*894–903, 1987.

Chapter 5

ECONOMICS OF MANAGED MENTAL HEALTH*

Richard G. Frank and Judith R. Lave

M anaged care is one of the fastest growing health submarkets in the United States. Although estimates of its size vary widely, (because there is no standard definition of managed care and little data) all observers agree that it is growing at a phenomenal rate. The Institute of Medicine (1989) defines utilization management "as a set of techniques used on or behalf of purchasers of health benefits to manage health care costs by influencing patient care decision making through case-by-case assessments of the appropriateness of care prior to its provision." The Institute estimates that there are over 250 organizations (most of which were established in the 1980s) that provide utilization management services for health plans that cover over 40 million people.

Historically, mental health accounted for roughly five to ten percent of expenditures made under private health insurance plans.[1] In recent years, however, such claims have been increasing more rapidly than for other health services. Current estimates indicate that from 10 to 30 percent of private health insurance payments are now made for mental health services (APA, 1988a).[2] The growing share of health insurance expenses claimed by mental health services has encouraged payors[3] to direct special attention to controlling their utilization.

This chapter explores the promise and the pitfalls of managed care as a method for controlling mental health utilization and costs within the context of private health insurance. It begins by discussing the tradi-

---

*This research was supported by grant #43703 from the National Institute of Mental Health

1. See APA (1988a,b), Wells et all (1982) and Frank and McGuire (1986) for some evidence on this issue.

2. There is a great deal of controversy as to what the actual level of growth in mental health expenditures has been. However, most observers agree that growth rates have accelerated in recent years. This has been attributed by some to significant growth in use of substance abuse services and inpatient care for mentally ill children and adolescents.

3. The term "payors" refers to the employers who offer health insurance as a fringe benefit, and to the insurance companies or the third party administrators that "manage" the health benefit.

tional "demand side" approaches to controlling mental health utilization—
the setting of limits on coverage and the imposition of high coinsurance.
It also reviews some "supply side" approaches—in particular, the implementation of prospective payment. The first of these has the effect of
withdrawing insurance coverage from people regardless of their need,
whereas the second contains incentives for under treatment. The chapter
goes on to discuss why managed care arrangements such as prior
authorization, concurrent review and case management of high-cost
patients could potentially control utilization and at the same time match
the clinical circumstances of individual patients with appropriate and
efficient treatment plans. The problems with implementing a managed
care approach are then outlined. Finally, the desirability and likelihood
of regulation of the managed care industry are examined.

Historical Approaches to Cost Control in Mental Health

The traditional approach to controlling expenditures for mental health
services under private health insurance plans has been to limit coverage.
In general, private insurance coverage for mental health is much more
restrictive than for other health care.

A 1986 Bureau of Labor Statistics (BLS) survey of employee benefits
found that only 37 percent of the health insurance plans offered by U.S.
employers had identical hospitalization coverage for mental as compared with non-mental health conditions; only six percent had identical
outpatient coverage for mental health and non-mental health. Coverage
for mental health and general health varies along a number of dimensions.
Private health insurance plans, for example, are likely to have much
stricter limits on coverage for both inpatient and outpatient mental
health services. Limits are expressed in either units of service and/or
dollars. Thus, 38 percent of plans surveyed by the BLS had limits on the
number of inpatient days covered while 33 percent limited the number
of outpatient visits; 26 percent of the plans had limits on expenditures
for inpatient services while 68 percent limited outpatient expenditures.
Cost sharing was higher for mental health services as well. While the
typical private health insurance plan has a coinsurance rate of 20 percent
for outpatient medical care, 48 percent of the plans surveyed had a 50
percent coinsurance rate for outpatient mental health services (APA
1988a).

One reason that cost sharing is higher for outpatient mental health services is that the use of such services is viewed as being more discretionary than for general medical care. There are two dimensions to this discretion: (1) Consumer demand for services is more discretionary, and (2) there is more discretion in the types of services used to treat a given problem. This view is supported by a number of studies done by economists to estimate the price elasticity of the demand for mental health services, or the extent to which the use of services varies with out-of-pocket costs.[4] While these studies differ considerably with regard to the populations studied and methods used, they consistently found that the use of outpatient mental health services was significantly more responsive to cost sharing arrangements than the use of outpatient medical services (Frank and McGuire, 1986; McGuire, 1981; Ellis and McGuire, 1986a; Horgan, 1986; Taube, Burnse and Kessler, 1986; and Keeler, 1988). Ellis (1986) extended this work by examining the effect of coverage limits (maximum expenditure provisions) on the use of mental health care. He found considerable response in demand for services to the coverage limit.

The reasons for setting limits on inpatient mental health coverage are somewhat different from outpatient care. High users of inpatient services tend to be severely and/or chronically mentally ill. Caring for the chronically mentally ill has traditionally been viewed as a public responsibility and virtually all states directly provide inpatient mental health care and some community services for them. Consequently, private plans often limit coverage, knowing that the enrollees are not totally without recourse. Limits may also be used because there is often honest disagreement on how to treat a particular case on an inpatient basis. Insurers may decide that they only want to provide insurance coverage for the less time intensive treatments.

There has been little research on the effect of cost sharing and benefit limits on the use of inpatient mental health services for people covered by private insurance. There has been research on the effect of limits for Medicaid patients. However, limits for public patients can be considered a supply side policy because providers cannot charge patients for extra days; limits for private patients are demand side policy because theoretically the patients could choose to stay in the

---

4. The term used for this in the insurance industry is "moral hazard." If the presence of insurance influences the behavior of the insured, "moral hazard" is said to exist.

hospital longer and pay for the extra days. The general impression, however, is that the limits are effective in controlling length of stay. Frank and Lave (1989) have studied the effect of limits on the length of stay of Medicaid patients. They were found to be effective in reducing the length of stay.

There are, however, two major problems with the strategy of using cost sharing and coverage limits to control utilization and costs. First, while this strategy does decrease utilization, it is not clear that it does so by reducing the use of the less effective services. For instance, research conducted by the RAND (Wells et al, 1982) corporation suggests that increased cost sharing reduces both "appropriate" and "inappropriate" use of services equally. The question is: if the use of services is lower with high cost sharing than it is with low, what services will not be received? Ideally, cost sharing should encourage people to be more thoughtful about when to seek services, to not seek care for trivial purposes or in cases when an interaction with a physician will make no difference such as for a head cold and to seek care when it has a higher probability of influencing health status. Second, these policies defeat, in part, one of the purposes of insurance which is to protect against low probability, but high cost events. Some of the people whose use exceeds the coverage limits will be liable for catastrophic costs.

In recent years, health plans have begun to change the way they pay providers in order to create incentive structures that promote the efficient delivery of services. These changes include the development of alternatives to the strict fee for service system (i.e., health maintenance organizations and preferred provider organizations) as well as changes in the way that traditional providers are paid for delivering services.

The most significant change in payment systems has been the development of prospective payment mechanisms for inpatient care. As a cost-containment strategy, this approach relies upon financial pressures to encourage clinical decision makers to be economical in their use of inpatient services. The most common type of prospective payment system is one in which hospitals are paid a prospectively determined amount for each discharge. The Medicare program adopted this general approach with the implementation of their prospective payment system, although all psychiatric hospitals and some general hospital psychiatric units have been exempted from the system (Lave et al., 1988).[5] In addition, several state Medicaid programs and a number of states that regulate hospital rates have also adopted per case prospective payment systems.

Research on the impact of per case prospective payment indicates that it leads to significant reductions in utilization of inpatient psychiatric care compared to the lengths of stay that would be expected under cost based payment methods with no limits (Freiman et al., 1989; Frank and Lave, 1989, 1986; Lave et al., 1988). The Medicaid program often places limits on the number of covered days. In these programs, the limits should be considered to be supply side policies since the hospitals cannot bill the Medicaid recipient for uncovered days. Under private insurance schemes, these limits are considered to be demand side policies since hospitals can bill private patients for uncovered days. In addition, studies of the impact of Medicare's prospective payment system and research on Medicaid payment methods (Lave and Frank, 1990) show that the treatment of psychiatric patients is more influenced by the payment method than is the treatment of patients with medical conditions. Although most of the studies reported to date were based on analyses of responses under public programs, the results suggest that use of prospective payment would be an effective means of reducing inpatient use of psychiatric care under private insurance schemes. This assumes that there are no offsetting increases in admissions for inpatient care. The research on this issue is mixed. Lave et al. (1988) found no evidence of significant increases in readmissions following adoption of prospective payment. In contrast Rupp, Steinwachs and Salkever (1984) report some increase in readmissions attributable to Maryland's prospective payment system.

As with the demand side, there are problems with these supply side policies. In particular, if there are incentives to reduce utilization, there are also incentives to under treat patients (Frank and Lave, 1986); Ellis and McGuire, 1989). Some have suggested that providers will be more likely to respond to the incentives to under treat when caring for the

---

5. Although psychiatric hospitals and some psychiatric units in general hospitals are exempt from the Medicare DRG based prospective payment system, they are not exempt from limits on payments. In general, Medicare reimburses these hospitals their average incurred costs per case — but there is a limit to the payment which is related to the provider's cost per case in a base year, indexed forward by a politically determined rate of increase. If the actual costs are less than this limit, the providers receive some incentive payments. The efficiency incentives embedded in this payment scheme are similar to those in prospective payment.

least articulate and most vulnerable patients such as the chronically and severely mentally ill.

The traditional approach to cost containment relies on very powerful tools: consumer cost sharing, limits on coverage and prospective payment for providers. The tools are quite effective in limiting utilization of mental health services. As noted, however, cost sharing and coverage limits reduce the level of insurance coverage. These strategies reduce the gains from risk spreading for which insurance is created in the first place. Policies aimed at influencing provider behavior through prospective payment have the advantage of not placing the burden of cost containment on psychiatric patients who are often vulnerable (McGuire, 1989). However, the incentives contained in payment systems such as per case prospective payment that successfully reduce utilization also reward under treatment. The traditional approach to cost containment also creates incentives to shift patients to the public sector.

The undesirable consequences of both cost sharing and payment policies have to do with how inclusive they are. They are applied to everyone, from the worried well to the very sick. Traditional cost-containment policies in private insurance plans do not generally recognize important differences in the clinical circumstances of individual patients nor do they take into account the availability of lower cost treatment alternatives. Per case prospective payment creates an incentive for a brief inpatient admission for a patient who might be just as well served by outpatient treatment. Approaches to cost containment that recognize heterogeneity and help patients negotiate what is often a complex and fragmented system of care offer an attractive alternative approach.

The Promise of Managed Care

Managed care represents an attempt to bring utilization under control. It is meant to evaluate the clinical circumstances of individual patients and constrain utilization to appropriate levels,[6] and to divert patients from high to lower cost treatment where outcomes will not be compromised by the shift. If traditional cost containment measures can be characterized as "sledge hammers," managed care promises to be a "scalpel."

The core techniques for managing care are prior authorization review, concurrent utilization review and high-cost case management. The empiri-

---

6. As will be discussed below the meaning of appropriate is critical and different parties have varying views on what level of use is appropriate.

cal basis for expecting that these techniques could be effective comes from a large set of studies that indicate: (1) there is a great deal of inappropriate care provided; (2) there is wide variation in treatment patterns for given types of psychiatric problems; (3) lengths of stay can be reduced in experimental settings without negatively influencing outcomes; (4) cost-effective alternatives to hospitalization exist; and (5) a small proportion of individuals account for a high proportion of ambulatory visits.

Several studies have been conducted to determine the appropriateness of hospital admissions and lengths of stay. Using specific clinical criteria, the researchers determined whether or not patients needed to be in hospitals. Although most of this research has focused on general medical and surgical cases, there have been a few studies of psychiatric cases. The conclusion of this body of research is that about 20 percent of inpatient days were inappropriate.

After controlling for insurance status, there is wide variation in the length of stay of patients with similar mental health diagnoses (Frank and Lave, 1985; Goldman, Taube and Jancks, 1987). As with other health conditions, lengths of stay for psychiatric disorders are consistently shorter in the Western region of the United States than they are in the East (Frank & Lave, 1986). Although part of this variation is probably due to unmeasured differences in the clinical condition of patients, much of it is the result of differences in "practice style." In addition, there is no apparent difference in the outcomes associated with these different lengths of stay. Thus, it seems possible that concurrent review could lead to decreases in lengths of stay.

There have been a number of controlled experiments in which investigators examined the effect of dramatically decreasing the length of stay (see Hargreaves and Shumaway, 1989, for a recent review). The majority of these studies were done in the 1970s when standard lengths of stay were long and when the experimental lengths of stay were closer to today's average. Nevertheless, the general conclusion of these studies was that reduced lengths of stay resulted in outcomes that were at least as good as those achieved for patients receiving extended inpatient care. These studies, however, do not inform us on several key questions related to managed care such as: What are the implications for patient outcomes of reducing stays below 1990 levels? For which patients can stays be most successfully reduced? Which types of patients need prolonged hospitalization? What specific technologies allow one to most effectively shorten hospital stays for psychiatric patients? Work by Talbott and Glick (1986) suggests that extended stays are appropriate for certain classes of severely mentally ill patients. This view is, however, quite controversial and has been challenged by Hargreaves and Shumway (1989).

There have been a number of studies that examined alternatives to inpatient hospitalization. (See Braun et al., 1981; Kiesler, 1982; Hargreaves and Shumway, 1989, for reviews.) These studies are relevant for evaluating the potential effectiveness of prior authorization certification and high cost case management.

There are three basis alternatives to inpatient psychiatric care: residential care, partial hospitalization and aggressive case management. Research on the effectiveness of residential alternatives to inpatient psychiatric care is decidedly mixed. A number of studies were not based on controlled experiments and so it is difficult to interpret their (generally positive) findings. The findings of studies that were based on an experimental design are also mixed. A number of controlled and quasi-experimental studies of partial hospital (or day care) programs were conducted in the 1960s and early 1970s. These early studies of day treatment suggested that, for significant segments of individuals at high risk of hospitalization, day treatment could serve as a successful alternative (Zwerling and Wilder, 1964). The results of more recent studies are more equivocal. Although they find that there are few significant differences in outcomes between hospitalized and day treatment patients (for example, Herz et al., 1971), the patient populations studied in these research efforts were very narrowly defined. The vast majority of patients typically referred to the experimental programs was "screened out" (for example, 78% of patients referred to the Herz et al. study were excluded). In sum, the evidence is weakly supportive of the notion that outcomes between day treatment and hospital care are comparable for some select psychiatric patients.

There have been a variety of studies of aggressive outreach programs and mobile treatment programs for community care of the severely mentally ill (the work of Stein and Test 1989 is perhaps best known). These studies took place in the context of a public system. While the results are generally quite favorable, the extent to which such technologies lend themselves to the context of private insurance is not clear.

Research on patterns of service utilization is relevant to the potential of case management to control high costs. Researchers have found that roughly 10% of the users of mental health care generate 50% of the expenditures (Taube et al., 1988). One third of these high users (or 3.3% of the population) were disabled and had multiple medical problems. This population was also far more likely to have used inpatient mental health services than were low users of outpatient mental health care. The research also indicated out that there was considerable heterogeneity among the high users of outpatient care. These findings suggest that there is potential for large savings (on the order of 15% to 20%) if the utilization of care by individuals without severe conditions is carefully controlled. This estimate is based on reducing use by the 66% of the high users who are not severely impaired to the average use levels of users of mental health care with characteristics that are similar to the "low disability" high users defined in the Taube et al. paper.

These research findings indicate that it should be possible to divert some patients away from costly inpatient care, to reduce the length of stay and to manage the care of high cost users of outpatient mental health care. It appears that managed care can lead to a more appropriate use of services for a given level of expenditures and limit costs more effectively than increased cost sharing or benefit limits. Prior authorization, concurrent review and high cost case management could lead to a more rational use of mental health services among those covered by private insurance.

The Pitfalls

There are a number of potential pitfalls in the application of managed care techniques to mental health. We classify these into four areas: (1) the organization and assumption of responsibility associated with managed care; (2) the clinical standards that form the basis for management; (3) the effectiveness of managed care; and (4) liability issues.

The Organization and Assumption of Responsibility

The American health care system is built upon a series of relationships in which one party acts on behalf of another. Economists refer to these as "agency" relations. Managed care arrangements alter some of these relationships in fundamental ways. In order for the new arrangements to be satisfactory, the roles, responsibilities and rights of each party must be redefined.

Figure 1 defines some of the key agency relationships. The rows represent parties who "hire" representatives to serve their interests in dealing with the health care system, while the columns identify those who serve as representatives (or agents) of the parties listed in the rows. The X's identify key agency relationships. Thus, patients hire physicians to provide care but also to serve as consultants to help "manage" their health problems and help resolve them. This advisory role constitutes the agency relationship.

Figure 1
Agency Relations

	Employer	Provider	Insuror	Care Manager
Employee	X		X	
Patient		X	X	X
Employer			X	X
Insuror				X

Managed care organizations are identified as agents for employers and insurers. The primary agency relationship, however, is with the employer. We consider the managed care organization as the agent whose role is to insure that the health care contract between the employer and the employee is enforced. This follows from the Institute of Medicine (1989) definition of utilization management as "Utilization management is a set of techniques used *by or on behalf of the purchaser* to manage health care decision making through case-by-case assessments of the *appropriateness* of care prior to its use" (emphasis added). The managed care organization can be viewed as having an agency relationship with employees as well since it provides information to help them make decisions.

Managed care arrangements interfere with the other agency arrangements. By definition, managed care reviews, monitors and makes judgments about whether the advice given by clinicians to their patients constitutes "medically necessary care." In order to determine whether managed care programs are desirable, however, it is necessary to know whether they lead to an overall increase in the effectiveness of the care and the efficiency with which it is provided. This line of argument presumes that patients do not have adequate information or make informed choices. The physician (or other provider) is hired to provide the information and serve as a consumer advocate. This weakening of the agency relationship also weakens the advocacy function. The result may be that less medical care is used than would be demanded by a fully-informed patient.

Managed care arrangements also change the relationship between the employer and the employee. The employer provides health insurance that promises to pay for "high-quality medically necessary" care. Inserting a managed care organization into this relationship may alter the terms of the contract between the employee and the employer. The managed care organization may enact standards that deviate from an implicit under-standing of what had previously been considered "high quality" and "necessary." The result may be that employees come to view their con-tracts with both their employer and insurer as having been violated. Disappointment, distrust and problems in the overall relationship may be the result.

The major point here is that the introduction of managed care may further complicate a set of already complex relationships. It is therefore critical to determine who the managed care organization really repre-sents and what its responsibilities are with regard to the interests of all the affected parties.

Clinical Standards

In order to properly implement managed care, protocols must be developed to guide the activity and a decision made about whether these should be made available to the providers. Those who manage care must have some basis on which to make judgments. If they are to decide whether care is appropriate, then some definition of appropriateness is necessary. It may, however, be more difficult to develop such definitions in mental health because there often are many theories on how to treat a given patient. According to Wells and Brook,

> Historical disagreement over the definition of mental health problems, treatment, and outcomes has made it difficult to develop the consensus required to develop specific criteria. . . . Providers that develop mental health services are diverse and have different assessment and treatment methods and priorities. Such diversity has complicated the develop-ment of criteria and standards. (Wells and Brook, 1989, p. 215.)

According to Gottlieb (1989), "The incentives of the mental health care system are confused by factors that may not affect general health care: controversial definitions of illness, poor standardization of triage and clinical decision making, a large variety of intervention strategies and a few gold standards of outcome" (p.225).

Given this diversity, it is not clear which standards should be used in developing the protocols for guiding managed mental health organizations. Most of them appear to base their protocols on "the community standard of care" (Institute of Medicine, 1989), and it is not clear what is to be done if there are many such standards. Consequently, it is not surprising that one of the more controversial aspects of managed care in mental health has to do with the clinical standards that are adopted for making prior authorization or concurrent review decisions (Ready, 1989).

Another controversial issue that must be addressed is whether the protocols, once developed, should be made public. Providers and patients argue that they should be able to evaluate and challenge the degree to which the decisions based on these protocols are "reasonable" and consistent with good clinical care. On the other hand, the managed care organizations argue that their criteria are proprietary and that if they distribute them, providers will be better able to "game" the system.

Given these complexities, it is not surprising that hospitals, physicians and other providers who interact with managed care organizations state that these organizations do not have clear standards for defining "appropriate care." It is also not surprising that the providers claim the standards are applied in an inconsistent manner (Mullen, 1989).

The Effectiveness of Managed Care

There has been very little research on the effectiveness of managed mental health. Utilization management is a new activity and most of the research on its effects has focused on general health care. While the federal government mandated Medicaid and Medicare to conduct peer review in the early 1970s, it was not until 1979 that CHAMPUS (health insurance for military dependent) adopted such a policy (Bassuk, undated). The early studies of some Professional Standards Review Organizations in the 1970s suggested that continued stay certification programs did not generate enough savings to pay for themselves (Averill and McMahan, 1977). More recently, Feldstein and colleagues (1988) analyzed all health care claims for an insurer that did not use prior authorization for all enrollees. Holding constant a number of relevant covariants, the authors found that managed care had a modest one time impact on expenditures although no significant effect on growth of expenditures was obtained. Careful analyses of managed care approaches in mental health are needed.

Thus, there remains a great deal of uncertainty about whether managed mental health programs are effective. It is important to conduct research on this issue, since the implementation of managed care techniques is costly. Not only are there costs incurred by the managed care company, but also there are additional costs to providers. Hospitals and other providers must hire people to interact with the reviewers who call about specific patients. In cases where the managed care company recommends a course of treatment different from that of the clinician, the clinician must interact with the company directly. Where there are real or potential denials, lawyers may be consulted.

Liability Issues

When important fiduciary relationships are altered without clear definitions of the rights and responsibilities of all parties, conflicts must often be resolved through the legal system. Some recent case law has begun to clarify some managed care issues. In *Sarchett* vs. *Blue Shield of California* (1989), for example, the State Supreme Court upheld the right of Blue Shield to challenge a physician's decision. Nevertheless, the opinion stated that ambiguities and uncertainties in a health insurance policy will be viewed in favor of the insured. Other case law already exists and is likely to grow rapidly.

Using the tort system to resolve such disputes can be inefficient. It is often a costly means for resolving conflict and standard of proof requirements discourage injured parties from pursuing recourse. If causation is difficult to establish, for example, injured parties may view the value of legal action as highly doubtful. Therefore, replacing a set of institutions where rights and responsibilities are relatively well defined with managed care arrangements and relying on the tort system to define rights and resolve disputes may not be socially desirable.

Regulation and Managed Care

Economists have long studied the conditions under which various organizational and contractual arrangements are likely to be efficient. If applied to managed care, a main conclusion of such work would likely be as follows: if rights are clearly defined, and can be traded; and if transaction costs are low, then managed care arrangements are likely to be efficient. That is, allowing managed care organizations to have a free hand in setting and administering standards would be efficient (see the work of Coase, 1960 and Farrell, 1987 for a detailed explanation of this conclusion).

It is likely, however, that the conditions set forth above will not be fulfilled. Two conditions in particular are likely to be problematic. First, it is our impression that the rights of various parties regarding receipt and payment for health services are not sufficiently well defined under many managed care arrangements. To some extent this is a problem in the original health insurance contract. Rights to challenge decisions by managed care organizations are often not clear (and have been brought to the courts on a number of occasions). The validity of the standards used may not be clear or open to the scrutiny of all parties involved in the arrangements. Medical necessity is a very elusive concept and definitions vary widely. This makes defining rights difficult in general and particularly so in mental health. An associated difficulty relates to defining the rights of patients and their financial liabilities when conflict arises between providers and managed care organizations.

Another efficiency condition likely to be violated has to do with transaction costs. If the tort system is relied upon to define rights and to impose penalties when rights are violated, then managed care organizations must in fact be penalized when this occurs. But it may be difficult to accomplish this because of the problems in establishing causation. Causation is usually the most difficult barrier for a plaintiff to overcome. The existing cases suggest that the provider has the burden of responsibility to contest decisions where there is disagreement with the managed care organization. This case law does not, of course, inform us on how to resolve situations where protests are lodged and how to assign liability if harm occurs subsequent to such a protest. For these reasons it may not be satisfactory to any of the parties—patients, insurers, employers, managed care organizations or society at large—to rely solely on the tort system.

An alternative would be to combine some public regulation with the tort system. Regulation could be used to lower the cost of resolving disputes by outlining a set of procedures that would define methods for setting and communicating review standards, specify formal steps for challenging and reviewing decisions made by managed care organizations and, where conflicts arise, define the rights and liabilities of patients. Steps toward such regulation, by several states and by managed care organizations themselves, are underway.

Conclusions

Expenditures for mental health services under private health insurance plans have been increasing more rapidly than for any other health services. It is therefore likely that payors will seek ways to control these expenditures. One option that they are considering in increasing numbers is managed care.

We believe that managed mental health care does offer some promise as a method for controlling the utilization and cost of mental health services. Ideally, utilization management could be used as a substitute for or complement to coverage limits as a method for insuring that the highest cost resources are targeted to the sickest patients. However, enough convincing data on the effectiveness of utilization management in mental health are not yet sufficiently available. It is therefore important that utilization management be evaluated. It is necessary that the savings from managed care more than offset its cost.

Managed care interferes with some well established relationships. It is important that those who interact with managed care organizations understand the way they function as well as the rights and the responsibilities of all the parties. These should be clearly specified. The basic standards used by these organizations should be public information. If the roles, responsibilities and obligations of all the parties to managed care are not well defined, there will be strong pressure for regulation.

Managed care, however, can be only one of the tools in the cost-containment toolbox. It is most likely to be effective in reducing the cost of selected high cost cases either by eliminating some unnecessary care or by diverting patients to less costly settings. The traditional tools of coverage limits, payment policies and cost sharing will continue to be important.

REFERENCES

American Psychiatric Association: *The Coverage Catalogue.* Washington, D.C., APA Press, 1988a.

American Psychiatric Association: *Eco-Facts, 1,* 1988b.

Averill, R.F., and McMahon, L.F.: A Cost benefit study on continued stay certification. *Medical Care, 15:*158–172, 1977.

Braun, P., Kochansky G., Shapiro R., et al.: Overview: Deinstitutionalization of psychiatric patients, a critical review of outcome studies. *American J. Psychiatry, 138*(6):736–749, 1981.

Coase R.: The problem of social cost. *J. of Law and Economics,* 3(1):1–44, 1960.

Ellis, R.P.: Strategic behavior in the presence of coverage ceilings and deductibles. *Rand J. Economics, 17*(2):158–175, 1986.

Ellis, R.P., and McGuire, T.G.: Cost sharing and patterns of mental health utilization. *J. Human Resources, 21*(3):359–380, 1986.

Farrell J.: Information and the coase theorem. *J. Economic Perspectives, 1*(2):113–129, 1987.

Feldstein, P.J., Wickizer, T.M., and Wheeler J.: The effects of utilization review programs on health care use and expenditures. *New England J. Medicine,* May 19, 1988, 1310–1314.

Frank, R.G., and Lave, J.R.: The psychiatric DRGs: Are they different? *Medical Care, 23*(11):1148–1155, 1985.

Frank, R.G., and Lave, J.R.: The effect of benefit design on the length of stay of Medicaid psychiatric patients. *Journal of Human Resources, 21*(3):321–337, 1986.

Frank, R.G., and Lave, J.R.: A comparison of hospital responses to reimbursement policies for medicaid psychiatric patients. *Rand J. Economics, 20*(4):588–600, 1989.

Frank, R.G., and McGuire, T.G.: A review of studies of the impact of insurance on the demand and utilization of specialty mental health services. *Health Services Research, 21:*241–266, 1986.

Goldman, H.H., Taube, C.A., and Jencks, S.F.: The organization of the psychiatric inpatient services system. *Medical Care, 25*(9):56–521, 1987.

Gottleib, G.L.: Diversity, uncertainty, and variations in practice: The behaviors and clinical decision making of mental health care providers. In Taube, C.A., Mechanic, D., and Hohnmann, A.A., (Eds): *The Future of Mental Health Services Research,* Washington, D.C., USGPO, 1989.

Hargreave, W.A., and Shumwag, M.: Effectiveness of mental health services for the severely mentally ill. In Taube, C.A., Mechanic, D., and Hohmann, A.A., (Eds.): *The Future of Mental Health Services Research,* Washington, D.C., USGPO, 1989.

Herz, M.I., Endicott, J., Spitzer, R.L. and Mesinkoff, A.: Day versus inpatient hospitalization: A controlled study. *American J. Psychiatry, 127*(10):107–117, 1971.

Horgan, C.M.: The demand for ambulatory mental health services from specialty providers. *Health Services Research,* 21:291–320, 1986.

Institute of Medicine: *Controlling Cost and Changing Patient Care.* Washington, D.C., NAS Press, 1989.

Keeler, E.B., Manning, W.G., and Wells K.B.: The demand for episode of mental health services. *Health Economics, 7*(4):369–392, 1988.

Keisler, C.A.: Mental hospitals and alternative care: Noninstitutionalization as potential public policy for mental patients. *American Psychologist, 37*(4):349–360, 1982.

Lave, J.R., Frank, R.G., Taube, C.A., et al.: PPS and psychiatry: The first year. *Inquiry, 25*(3):354–363.

Lave, J.R., and Frank, R.G.: The effect of the structure of hospital payment on length of stay. *Health Services Research, 25*(2), 1990.

McGuire, T.G.: *Financing Psychotherapy.* Cambridge, Ballinger, 1981.

McGuire, T.G.: Financing and reimbursement of mental health services. In Taube, C.A., Mechanic, D., and Hohmann, A.A., (Eds): *The Future of Mental Health Services Research,* Washington, D.C., USGPO, 1989.

Stein, L.I., and Test, M.A.: Alternative to mental hospital treatment: conceptual model treatment program and clinical evaluation. *Archives of General Psychiatry, 37:*392–397, 1980.

Taube, C.A., Kessler, L.G., and Burns, B.J.: Estimating the probability and level of ambulatory mental health use. *Health Services Research, 21:*321–340, 1986.

Taube, C.A., Goldman, H.H., Burns B.J., et al.: High users of outpatient mental health services I: Definition and characteristics. *American J. Psychiatry, 145*(1):19–24, 1988.

Wells, K.B., Manning, W.G., Duan, N., et al.: *Use of Ambulatory Mental Health Care.* Santa Monica, The Rand Corporation, 1982.

Wells, K.B. and Brook R.H.: The quality of mental health services: Past, present and future. In Taube, C.A., Mechanic, D., and Hohmann, (Eds): *The Future of Mental Health Services Research,* Washington, D.C., USGPO, 1989.

Zwerling, I. and Wilder, J.F.: An evaluation of the applicability of the day hospital in treatment of acutely disturbed patients. *Israel Annals of Psychiatry and Related Disciplines, 2:*162–185, 1964.

Chapter 6

MANAGED MENTAL HEALTH: THE INSURER'S PERSPECTIVE

Richard Kunnes

During the past decade, costs for mental health and substance abuse services have increased dramatically. Unfortunately, there is no evidence to suggest that the increase in services provided or money paid have resulted in any improvement in quality. In fact, there may well be a decline in quality due to overutilization, consequent increases in patient dependence, and decreases in patient adaptability (Mullen, 1989). What are the factors that have led to this frustrating dilemma?

Unmet Need and Lessening of Stigma

There is mounting evidence that debilitating psychiatric and substance abuse disorders affect as much as 20 percent of the general population, yet only a small fraction receive relevant cost- and quality-effective care (Thomas, 1990). Such unmet needs do not, of themselves, mean that the rapid expansion in the utilization of psychiatric and substance abuse services is a positive development. It simply suggests, among many other things, that there is a "tappable" well, that a number of psychiatric and substance abuse providers have hit a gusher, and an expanding number of others hope to be as lucky (Chasnoff, 1988).

In the past, when one had a psychiatric and/or substance abuse disorder, the stigma was such that treatment was avoided altogether, or received only in the most isolated of settings, e.g., from "snake pits" to hot springs (Fry, 1989). Stigma, at least for substance abuse, has been turned on its head and replaced by "glamourization." One need only glance at the celebrity parade of visible patients to be aware that there is sometimes as much raw clinical data in the *National Enquirer* as in the *New England Journal of Medicine.* When both Betty Ford and Kitty Dukakis are praised for their efforts toward destigmatization, a veritable bipartisan coalition for fixed-day inpatient treatment is established.

Grateful Acknowledgment. Gary Whitted, Ph.D., Director of Health Cost Containment, The Travelers Companies, significantly contributed to many of the concepts in this chapter.

101

Shift in Responsibility

The shift toward "psychiatricization" of problems that are as much social and/or legal has provided a huge pool of new "patients" (Bryant, 1990; Darton, 1989). This is particularly true for adolescents (Krantz, 1990; Fink, 1989). Adjustment and conduct disorders, drug/alcohol experimentation, sexual discomforts and religious fundamentalism (including cultism), for example, are especially relevant to adolescents and have been seized upon by inpatient programs, aware that many such adolescents have significant inpatient insurance benefits (Kim, 1988; Droste, 1988).

The same dynamic is apparent in court-mandated drunk driving treatment programs. Inevitably, the mandate is inpatient treatment, not just treatment, but also implicitly for punishment and incarceration as well. The inpatient setting will often perform neither function very well, at least not as well as others can.

Expansion of Insurance Benefits

The increase in benefits for inpatient psychiatric and substance abuse disorders has led to increased inpatient utilization, facilitated in part by increases in mandated benefits. Benefits are not only being increased by legislatures and regulatory entities but by the courts as well. Class action suits demanding that certain psychiatric diagnoses (e.g., bipolar disorders, autism, etc.) be covered to the same extent as "physical" illness have taken place in several areas. And in at least one case, the plaintiff's position was supported. Increased benefits for psychiatric and substance abuse disorders, however, do not, by themselves cause increases in cost and decreases in the quality of care. Rather, the cost and quality problems are more directly tied to marketing that induces (and seduces) prospective patients and their referring practitioners to use their inpatient benefits. And in an environment of unmanaged services, liberal benefits will almost inevitably lead to unnecessary use, high costs, and questionable quality.

Inpatient Chains and Franchised Vendors

Most psychiatric and substance abuse beds are excluded from prospective payment systems, including federal DRGs (Levick, 1988). This has helped stimulate the conversion of medical/surgical beds to psychiatric and/or substance abuse use. And new hospitals have been built in record numbers—100 in 1988–1989 alone. In the same period, 100 medical/surgical facilities were closed. Many of the psych/substance abuse hospitals run at only 40%–50% occupancy. To increase utilization, their owners have created new markets and urge hospitalization for such disorders as religious and sexual addiction. While in some cases these may represent serious clinical problems, the overwhelming majority do not need acute inpatient treatment (Herrington, 1989; Pallarito, 1989).

One major chain has boasted that it would build and own, within two years, one psychiatric/substance abuse facility within two hours of every person in the United States (Mayer, 1989). Such franchising and other expansions of inpatient services have had a deleterious effect on insurance benefits. They are leading to overutilization, higher costs and payor motivation to decrease benefits. Associated with hospital chains and franchised care have been tremendous increases in television, radio, billboard and print advertising, a virtual "McDonaldization" of services (Gibson, 1989). One well-known substance abuse facility ran an advertisement (EAP Digest, 1989) directed toward employers noting that even "you" (Mr. or Ms. Employer) can "recognize trouble" by examining the provided "Hints of Trouble" list. The list is extremely broad and ambiguous. It includes, for example, behavior such as "long periods of time spent in the bathroom," "resentment toward authority," "sudden unfriendliness," "loss of ambition," and others. The implied solution for these "troubles" is hospitalization at the advertised facility. While such behavioral manifestations should not be ignored, to imply that hospitalization is the solution (if indeed a solution is even required) only adds to unnecessary inpatient utilization.

Incentives to Psychiatrists for Hospitalizing Patients

Within a very limited (and perhaps perverse) context, it is often more economically rewarding for psychiatrists to hospitalize their patients, rather than treating them on an outpatient basis. In the hospital, a lot of patients can be seen very quickly and the remuneration is substantial. So-called "wave therapy," where some psychiatrists, in effect, wave at their hospitalized patients, say, "Hi, how are you?" and charge for a full session for each patient is more factual than funny. Somewhat less egregious, some psychiatrists not uncommonly see their hospitalized patients back-to-back for 20–30 minutes each and charge for a full session in each case.

Some psychiatric hospitals offer psychiatrists a "bonus" for every 3–5 patients admitted, based either on the number of admissions or length of stay. These psychiatric "frequent flyer," profit-sharing arrangements are not always based on medical necessity (Prosser, 1989). When managed care-oriented psychiatrists attempt to lessen lengths of stay, some psychiatric hospitals have other staff encourage patients to stay longer (Tigner, 1989).

Benefit Plan Designs That Encourage Hospitalization

Traditional (and contrary to common sense) insurance benefit designs have encouraged inpatient and discouraged non-hospital services. Plans with 90–100% coverage for inpatient and 50–60% coverage for outpatient services inevitably and forcefully incentivize inpatient care. Those that do not provide coverage for partial care or do so at low rates further encourage the use of the most intensive care in the most expensive places. This has been particularly true in mental health and substance abuse, in spite of conclusive research and experience suggesting that such benefit designs are neither cost effective nor supportive of quality care.

Gross Over Utilization

The above factors have contributed to enormous overutilization of inpatient services. Many Fortune 500 companies are now experiencing psychiatric and substance abuse costs at a rate of 20% to 25% of their total health care costs (Mullen 1989), with an inflationary trend of 20–30% per annum. In 1989, the increase in mental health and substance abuse costs for companies with 5,000 or more employees was just under 50%! This trend far exceeds both the general and the medical and hospital consumer price index combined (Duva, 1989). Inpatient costs comprise 75–90% of the mental health and substance claim dollar. Even in health maintenance organizations (HMOs), considered the most stringently managed of all health care providers, there appears to be large waste and unnecessary utilization of inpatient mental health and substance abuse services (Paris, 1990).

In three HMOs owned by a major national insurance company, for example, utilization management and treatment service networks were installed. Prior to these, the HMOs had a three-tiered gatekeeping system for management of potential mental health and substance abuse acute hospitalization. The three tiers were the patient's primary care physician (PCP), the HMO's utilization review nurse, and the HMO's local medical director. Of these, none had used specialized mental health/substance abuse utilization management techniques in the past. It had been assumed that by requiring such a three-tiered approval, inpatient admissions would be kept to the bare minimum, i.e., only what was medically necessary. This was not the case and it was decided to implement a specialized utilization management system including a full treatment network *and* a full range of management and coordination techniques. Bed days per thousand HMO members per month were cut in half.

This new specialized management approach did not result in increased quality problems. There was no increase in patient grievances, no decrease in patient satisfaction ratings, no increase in red-flag/occurrence cases, and no increase in cases with less than optimal treatment, using the HMOs' *prior* standard of optimality (i.e., prior to the specialized utilization management system).

The success of such an approach in these HMOs, an already managed care environment, suggests a general level of hospital over-utilization for mental health and substance abuse within the general system of care throughout the country. Even within the narrow and stringently managed context of the HMO, there appears to be enormous over-utilization. This suggests a problem in the quality of those services if, in fact, they are not necessary (Shadle, 1989).

This is not to deny that those HMO members who were hospitalized unnecessarily needed help. In fact, every one of them had significant clinical syndromes in need of extensive clinical services. But they did not need inpatient care. And, in fact, these patients may have done much better, e.g., had a lower level of symptomatology achieved more quickly, had they been treated in other, less intense, settings.

RESPONSE OF THE INSURERS

Cutting Benefits

There are many approaches to cutting benefits (Chodoff, 1987). These include limitations on dollar and/or day (calendar or lifetime) amounts, higher deductibles, lower co-insurance coverage, no stop-loss applicability, no or minimal substance abuse benefits, no or minimal benefits for

dependents, and several others. These have been implemented in count-
less different arrangements (Bailey, 1989; Pereira, 1989). Some of the
disadvantages of this "scorched earth" approach are:

- Employee dissatisfaction (Firshein, 1990)
- Diagnosis gaming, e.g., treat alcoholism under a diagnosis of esopha-
  gitis or pancreatitis (Hellerstein, 1987)
- Significant delays in treatment with consequential and ultimate
  increases in treatment costs not only for mental health and sub-
  stance abuse disorders, but for physical disorders as well (Bruce,
  1989; Gelber, 1989).
- Increased staff turnover
- Increased disability or workers' compensation cost
- Increased costs for job training
- Higher absenteeism

Telephone Utilization Review

Many insurance carriers have invested heavily in telephone utilization review (UR) systems. While such an approach has cut some of
the extreme edges of inappropriate hospital utilization, the overall
impact is at best marginal (Brazda, 1990). Most UR measurements of
effectiveness report savings in the context of "days saved" measured
in two ways: comparing requested days to actual days, or comparing
national or regional average length of stay "norms" to actual days.
Both measurements are fairly soft. In the first, the more "sophisticated"
practitioners will inflate the number of days requested as a bargaining
hedge. In the second scenario, the national or regional "norm" may
have little or no relationship to the patient's benefit design or the
practitioner population with which the UR organization is working
(Vibbert, 1990). In either case, the so called "savings" may be non-
existent.

Telephone Case Management

This is an approach that is typically associated with telephone UR.
It usually involves those cases not successfully managed by the UR
organization, and where at least 15 to 30 days have elapsed since
admission. The standard mechanism is to negotiate with the treating
psychiatrist, the patient, the family and employer an "in lieu of"

hospitalization contract. Typically, the patient will have better inpatient benefits than other alternatives. In exchange for leaving the hospital, a non-hospital benefit will be provided at a higher than usual amount, one ordinarily available only for hospital coverage.

This approach can reduce some of the wider variations in utilization associated with long-term psychiatric hospitalization. In general, it has had little effect on fixed-day substance abuse treatment programs. This is true, in part, because many telephone case management programs don't "kick in" until 30 days have elapsed, and the fixed day programs are usually for 28-day stays. Here too, the reported savings are "soft." They tend to use a "what-would-have-likely-happened" approach, i.e., if this patient were not case managed and removed from the hospital, how many additional days *would* there have been?

Claims Management

Many insurance carriers are developing specialized claim units for mental health and substance abuse. These units have had some success — some of the extremes in billing have been reduced (Grumet, 1989). Savings here are based on claim reports long after someone has started or even completed treatment. Claims review is at best concurrent. More likely, it is retrospective, when the damage has already been done, and the bill must be paid. It is essentially claims management rather than care management.

Standard Preferred Provider Organizations

Standard preferred provider organizations (PPOs) usually have a full range of medical and surgical services and just a smattering of psychiatrists and psychiatric facilities. Many of them do not include mental health professionals other than psychiatrists or sub-specialists. Further, standard PPOs do not include a sufficient range of inpatient alternatives such as day treatment, half-way house and structured out-patient programs. These alternatives are crucial for cost-effective, quality care. Nor does the standard PPO have a local specialty-specific, management system able to match services with symptoms, routinely and effectively.

While standard PPOs can get some savings through discounted care, there is little evidence that significant savings are achieved for mental health and substance abuse services. This may be true for two reasons: first, they are less able to negotiate the type of volume-driven discounts that can be achieved by specialty PPOs; second, significant discounts alone, without stringent case management, may ultimately produce no savings if the discounts are simply compensated for by increased utilization.

Limitations

The above approaches have had a minimal effect on slowing the rate of inflation for mental health and substance abuse services. In this light, it is reasonable to ask why the major carriers continue with them. A major factor has been their overreliance on the prestige and perceived expertise of the medical profession combined with the belated recognition that mental health and substance abuse cannot be managed by the same methods as medical and surgical disorders (Traska, 1989; Gaver, 1988). And the perception that mental health and substance abuse services are grossly overused is relatively new. Although present for decades, it has generally been visible and "felt" only since the early 1980s.

The corporate cultures of the major insurance carriers have also contributed to their approaches to containing the costs of mental health and substance abuse services. They are among the largest, richest and most bureaucratically complex corporations in America. This has bred a culture of caution and conservatism. Some of this has been very healthy and appropriate to their financial and ethical responsibilities. But it also tends to cause them to equate the status quo with the state of the art.

Perhaps most important, the carriers are ultimately required to do the bidding of their corporate clients. These clients and their consultants have, for the most part, been every bit as conservative as the carriers. And, not infrequently, they have actively encouraged carrier passivity, even in the face of hemorrhaging claim dollars (Bureau of Labor Statistics, 1989). Thus, the cost-containment measures that have been used represent an accommodation to all the above corporate-client factors. They have tried to advance in small steps and in ways most familiar to all of the key parties.

But where are they going now? And why? It is becoming increasingly clear to them that what they have done so far has not worked, and that other approaches have been more successful. These include HMOs and community mental health centers (CMHCs), both of which have been around for decades (Herrington 1989; Brightbill, 1988). Further, carriers and others have been piloting specialized mental health and substance abuse HMO-type configurations since at least 1983, using many of the most successful, cost-effective techniques developed by CMHCs. Such approaches as 24-hour accessibility, triage and case management systems, use of social workers and psychologists, crisis intervention, day treatment and partial hospitalization, etc., are now at the heart of the carriers' cost-effective, specialized managed care programs (Whitted, 1989).

THE INSURER ADVANTAGE

The major insurance carriers now appear to acknowledge that the cost-effective coverage of mental health and substance abuse services requires a comprehensive approach that integrates a broad spectrum of programs, services and procedures. What follows is a discussion of what, from the carrier's perspective would be considered the components of an "ideal" system and the direction in which the managed mental health field seems to be moving.

National Networks

The quality and cost-effectiveness of a local managed care network is enhanced by others integrated with it on a regional or national scope. Many employers are regional or national and want to provide the same level and style of care for as many of their employees as possible. This can best be done by major national insurance companies with managed networks in at least 30–50 cities. Such networks allow for national standards and a three-tiered, cross-checking, mutually reinforcing quality assurance/utilization management system (Nissen, 1990).

Networks in multiple cities allow those rural areas, for example, to use more network cities as "centers of excellence" when specialized or inpatient care is required and not immediately available in outlying areas.

Multiple networks on a national basis allow for a greater range of administrative experimentation. The same specialty network in the same city, for example, may be used as the managed care network for all of an insurance company's products, e.g., HMOs, PPO, disability and worker's compensation, phone UR/case management, claims consultation and others.

Dedicated Telephone Units

A telephone system is needed that is national in scope and used solely for mental health and substance abuse utilization, triage and case management. The service must be staffed solely by registered psychiatric nurses, masters-level psychiatric social workers or psychologists, and fully supported by board-eligible or certified psychiatrist advisors. The system must be specialized in terms of major diagnostic areas, e.g., child, adolescent, adult, alcoholism/substance abuse, eating disorders, affective disorders, etc. The staff must be divided into these targeted, major diagnostic areas.

All service management functions, e.g., UR, triage and case management, must be integrated into a single prospective and concurrent comprehensive care management system. All cases must be managed, if possible, prior to the inception of treatment. The case management process must apply to inpatient and outpatient care and be supported by a high-tech claims review system.

The program should be nationally accessible 24 hours a day, seven days a week. It must be managed so that claim expense guarantees can offer substantial savings, many times greater than what it costs. Detailed written criteria and protocols for these services must be available with full staff orientation into this approach.

Specialty Claim Units

Nationally capable, high-tech, specialized and dedicated psychiatric and substance abuse claim units are also critical for concurrent and retrospective reviews of psychiatric and substance abuse claims that are either "non-compliant" (e.g., out-of-network, out-of-plan) or out-of-area (geographic).

These specialized claim units must also facilely perform bill audits for both outpatient and inpatient services, for psychiatric and/or substance abuse cases, and for children and adults, with sub-specializing psychiatric physician advisors.

EAPs

EAPs must be available to fill the geographic and service gaps, i.e., to be where integrated management and clinical networks are not. The EAP professionals must be carefully selected on the basis of successful experience in and commitment to cost effective, quality, managed care.

EAPs have traditionally not been part of the managed care scene (with some exceptions). They have significantly over-referred to fixed-day inpatient treatment programs, and have been as much a part of the overutilization problem as the solution. While the EAP marketplace is evolving toward a more managed context, careful selectivity for EAPs is key. If EAPs are to be involved, they must be not only the front line of but also the highly integrated partner in the management system (Brill, 1985).

Population Factors

In areas where geography and/or population size make impractical a full provider network, "mini-networks" can provide a high level of quality and cost-effective care. A local managed care oriented employee assistance program combined with a mandatory national telephone prospective case management system can be effective in lessening unnecessary hospitalization and increasing the quality of care.

This system is particularly enhanced when the benefit structure allows benefit substitution, e.g., two or three outpatient days for every inpatient day, where the locus and intensity of treatment is determined on the spot by a case manager, in consultation with the treating practitioner and board-certified psychiatric advisor.

Unified Approach

All of these services should be directed by a single, specialized administrative and clinical entity. Such an approach leads to greater consistency as well as a more uniform overall approach to services. The criteria used for all services, for example, should be the same, without regard to benefit design. This allows not only for greater ease of administration but also for greater equity among employees, wherever they live. A unified system allows for the same benefits, without regard to where people live. Any so-called out-of-network penalties would be assessed on the basis of compliance/non-compliance, not on the presence/absence of a network.

A unified system and strategy also allow for a higher level of quality, as quality standards, parameters, protocols and methods of evaluation will be virtually one and the same, without regard to where the patient lives, assuming benefit coverage and design are equivalent. This is not to say that a patient in a metropolitan network will receive exactly the same care as someone out of the network in a rural area. Rather, the methods for measuring, administering and determining the cost, quality and quantity of services should be basically the same throughout all services, systems and sites (Fauman, 1989).

One Stop Shopping

So-called "boutique" or "niche player" managed mental health companies, as opposed to major national insurance companies, have, as virtually their sole source of profits, the shared savings produced by decreasing treatment utilization. Having such shared savings as a primary source of their income incentivizes them both to underutilize (the most significant quality concern in the managed care setting) and to take a large (larger than a comprehensive insurance company would) share of the employer's saved claim costs. This leaves the employer with less money to enhance employee health benefits in other areas and is thus a potential quality and cost-effectiveness concern (Sack, 1989).

Further, because such niche players are, by definition, much smaller than the major insurance companies, they may not be able to provide state-of-the-art claim review systems, national prospective case management programs, and a national network of EAPs and providers. The one-stop shopping advantage of the major insurance company is exemplified by the breadth and depth of its integrated products and services, e.g., management, administration, human resources, clinical, insurance, technical consulting, claims, reporting, and marketing systems. These products and services allow for a much greater level of savings to be returned to the employer (due to diversified sources of carrier profits) and greater ease of administrative liaison and negotiations between client and carrier.

Benefit Coverage

Managed care has traditionally been associated with decreased benefits, particularly for mental health and substance abuse. This is particularly noticeable in standard indemnity plans as compared with HMO benefits (Coniaris, 1989). The managed care HMO benefits are customarily much lower than those in most indemnity plans.

To achieve high-quality, cost-effective mental health and substance abuse services, the managed care program must cover virtually all medically necessary services, exclude those that are not and limit freedom of provider choice. In effect, employee and employer agree to exchange a more limited choice of provider for increased coverage, increased quality and increased cost controls (White 1990; Altshuler, 1989). Failure to cover needed care results in more expensive care later on (Millman, 1989). It not only leads to increased psychiatric symptomatology, but to greater medical/surgical symptomatology and utilization as well (Freudenheim, 1989). This is particularly true for substance abuse. A number of studies have indicated that 45–55% of medical/surgical patients have associated alcoholism disorders (Brazda, 1989). Poor coverage leads to poor care and higher costs (Kim, 1989). Increasing benefits can lead to better care and lower costs, so long as care is provided in a highly managed program (Klerman, 1989).

Mandated Benefits

Insurance companies have traditionally been (and still are) strongly opposed to mandated benefits. This attitude may be counterproductive, particularly with mental health and substance abuse disorders, for the reasons stated above and others. Because overutilization is so rampant, billions of dollars are wasted on unnecessary services. These wasted dollars are recoupable in the context of simultaneously mandated *and* managed benefits, particularly with mental health and substance abuse disorders.

Increases in certain mandated benefits do not, themselves, cause increases in utilization and costs, if those mandated benefits are offered *only* in the context of a highly managed care setting (HIAA, 1989). Mandating an increase in inpatient benefits from 30 to 60 days, for example, will not increase utilization, if the benefit is managed properly. In fact, trading increased benefits for increased benefit management will decrease utilization and cost and improve quality (Bigelow, 1989).

The controls required to produce such a happy scenario are:

- A local, in-person, managed care network;
- At least a 20–30% coinsurance differential between in- and out-of-network services (i.e., in and out of compliance with case management recommendations) (DiBlase, 1989);
- Out-of-network claims or those out of compliance with prospective case management not applied to the stop loss;
- Out-of-network (or out-of-compliance) benefit maximums limited to a community average, e.g., $500 per diem for hospitalization. In a

typical "90-60" plan, i.e., 90% coverage for in-network services and 60% for out-of-network, the maximum claim payout for out-of-network would be $300 (60% × $500). This makes it unlikely that very expensive hospitals (those charging far more than $500) would accept the $300 as payment in full. They would impose a copayment on the patient and thus discourage the use of such hospitals;

• Out-of-network inpatient days beyond 30 must be approved by the insurance carrier's psychiatric director.

There are a number of other disincentives and mechanisms to discourage "leakage" out of the managed care system. Significant increases in outpatient coverage (especially to the point of parity with inpatient), may not only motivate patients to stay within the network but also to greater use of outpatient services (Marsh and McLennan, 1990).

Mandated benefits can be a disaster when they preclude significant differentials between in- and out-of-network care. The design of mandated benefits should include important incentives to stay in the system and strong disincentives to stray. If these incentives are not present, mandated increases in benefits will lead ineluctably to increased inapproprite utilization, poorer care and higher costs (Melnick, 1989). Where this happens, employers will ultimately cut benefits in other non-mandated areas and shift more and more costs to the employee. The result will discourage *both* necessary and unnecessary care.

Benefit Design

Benefit design in the context of a highly managed system should provide for both disease and intensity neutrality. Intensity neutrality means that the managed care system and benefit design should not encourage, for example, inpatient over outpatient over intermediate level care (e.g., day treatment). Unnecessary utilization of inpatient services, where outpatient is more appropriate, may result in increased patient dependency and recidivism, more disability and higher costs.

Disease neutrality requires that the benefits not encourage manipulation of diagnosis or treatment through differentiating between mental health and substance abuse disorders. From a clinical as well as a claims viewpoint it is difficult to tell which is the primary or secondary diagnosis more often than not. Virtually all substance abuse disorders, for example, have some elements of anxiety and depression (Bukstein, 1989). Poorer coverage for substance abuse than for mental disorders may cause a significant number of disorders for substance abuse to be treated as psychiatric. This could result in poor care and higher costs, given the increased risk of recidivism in such a scenario (Cresson, 1989).

Benefit differences between mental health and substance abuse on the one hand and medical/surgical disorders on the other, also do not lead to cost-effective or quality care. Benefits for mental health and substance abuse are often at subsistence levels compared with those for medical and surgical disorders. The alcoholic with poor substance abuse coverage who needs treatment, may have a "benign" family physician who will hospitalize the patient for "gastritis." Neither the "gastritis" nor the alcoholism will be adequately treated, resulting in increased utilization and costs (Connolly, 1988).

By carefully increasing *and* managing benefits, enormous amounts of wasted care can be avoided. One major insurance company estimates that 40% of inpatient psychiatric days are unnecessary as are 80–90% of post-detoxification inpatient days for substance abuse. Estimates are that even 30–40% of detoxification inpatient days are not medically necessary (Hayashida, 1989). These patients do have serious and even severe clinical syndromes but inpatient treatment is not required (Kenkel, 1990). With huge increases in their mental health and substance abuse costs, many employers are at a crossroads. They can either control costs by reducing coverage or they can increase coverage by limiting choice and managing care. Some of the more Draconian schemes call for cutting both choice and coverage (Howard, 1989).

THE SERVICE SYSTEM

The treatment network and the services it provides are, of course, central to the success of managed mental health care. From the insurance carrier's perspective, there are a number of elements that should be present in any effective service system.

Sole Entry Point

The patient should enter the managed care system only through an accessible 800 number. This number should be available 24 hours a day, seven days a week. There should be no other initial access point and attempts to access any other way may result in non-compliance penalties.

Where there is an employee assistance program (EAP), calls to the EAP should use the same method of access. Educating and obtaining the cooperation of the EAP is very important. Failure to integrate it with the managed care system may undermine its cost-effectiveness. Many EAP staff members are zealous advocates of fixed day inpatient programs. If they convey this commitment to patients, the stage is set for unnecessary inpatient utilization, particularly if the EAP is not a part of the managed care system (Bradman, 1989).

If the employer does not have an EAP and wants one, it should be provided by the managed care program and be part of the managed care network. A single entry point, i.e., the 800 number, also simplifies referrals to the system, whether they are self-referrals, EAP, or other. This is particularly helpful in emergency situations.

Triage

The 800 number should be answered by a triage professional who assesses the problems and arranges for help. This process of assessment and assignment is particularly important in emergency situations and the triage staff must be able to identify true emergencies (Rodin, 1989).

The true emergency should be assigned immediate and intensive face-to-face evaluation and treatment. In an acute emergency, a network psychiatrist should meet the patient at the nearest facility, usually within an hour. A less emergent situation may allow for the patient to go to a clinician's office six to eight hours later. All patients should be seen within 72 hours.

The triage professional has the initial responsibility by phone and face-to-face to match service needs with symptom acuity/functional risk. A mildly addicted, non-suicidal adolescent substance abuser of amphetamines, for example, would be given an early appointment with a clinician specializing in outpatient adolescent substance abuse detoxification and rehabilitation (Wright, 1989).

The face-to-face functional and mental status examination should produce sufficient clinical information to allow the triage professional to not only match symptoms with services, but to avoid unnecessary hospitalization. Once a patient is admitted to the hospital for whatever reason, a transfer to non-hospital programs is difficult, irrespective of how clearly unnecessary the hospitalization may be. To minimize unnecessary hospital utilization, the best approach is to avoid the admission in the first place, wherever possible (Kim, 1988). Avoiding unnecessary hospitalization is key to cost effectiveness. And without cost effectiveness, the employer will cut coverage and quality.

The triage system should be vertically and horizontally integrated to best match symptom acuity with service intensity. Cost-effective and vertically integrated triage and case management should make possible the broadest range of services, from most to least intense. Triage and case management should also be horizontally integrated, including the widest range of providers as part of the local service network. The system should have the ability to provide a wide variety of treatment modalities, including self-help groups (Klerman, 1987), intensive outpatient services and intermediate services as well (Herrington, 1989).

Emphasis on Alternatives to Inpatient Care

Intermediate level services should include such things as partial hospitalization, adult foster care, halfway and quarterway houses, adult and child day treatment, home care, and residential treatment (Glaser, 1989). Intensive outpatient care could be twice a day or five times a week. There are a wide variety of intensive outpatient treatment programs that are routinely ignored despite their effectiveness as an alternative to standard inpatient care (Gillig, 1989). Breadth and depth of services are essential to customize the network, individualize the services and assure cost effectiveness and quality.

Matching services with symptoms, e.g., individualizing treatment according to medical necessity and appropriateness, avoids a "cookie cutter" approach to treatment and increases the likelihood of a symptom-free and functional patient. Contrary to this approach are fixed day inpatient treatment programs. Such programs are the antithesis of individualized treatment. After all, how can all alcoholics require the same 28 days of treatment? Historically, the 28-day program was chosen primarily on the basis of benefit limits, not medical necessity or desirability.

Unnecessary confinement may seriously impair a patient's ultimate adaptability to everyday stress. Such confinements create and maintain an artificial, relatively low stress, dependency-inducing environment. They do not prepare a patient to function well at work or home. Miraculous "cures" can, and commonly do, become transformed into relapse and recidivism by the stresses and strains of everyday life—the street, work and home (Smith, 1989).

Clinically and financially sound treatment programs must prepare the patient for the highest level of independent functioning by providing treatment in the context of real-life stress (Droste, 1989). By avoiding fixed day treatment programs and limiting confinement to only what is necessary, independence of performance and overall functionality can be addressed and increased from the first day of treatment. They can also reduce absenteeism and enhance an early return to work and productivity. Overutilization of inpatient care is expensive, not just because of the treatment cost but because it may lead to poor stress adaptability and recidivism (Cavaini, 1990), increased time away from work, and increased disability and workers' compensation benefits (Donkin, 1989).

Quality Based on Function

In clinical settings, standards of quality have traditionally been based on diagnosis and conventional symptoms. While it is unreasonable to disregard this approach, it is necessary, from the insurance carrier's perspective, to modify it (Wells, 1989; Friedman, 1989). Insurance programs and their managed care components are commercial products sold to customers and must satisfy customer needs. It is not unreasonable to expect that the customer (employer) may be more interested in the overall functional performance of employees than in their feelings and symptoms, to the degree that these may be distinguishable. In this context, quality assurance must measure and enhance the requirement for healthy and functional employees. Changes in absenteeism, productivity, relationships with co-workers, substance abuse and other measures of function are important (Wenzel, 1988; Goering, 1988).

To enhance quality, there should be a wide range of closely coordinated services and settings. Services cannot be well coordinated unless they are continuously and unobtrusively managed. In effect, such functions as triage, case management, utilization review, discharge coordination, aftercare follow-up, etc., should be so self-contained that to both patient and provider, the service and management are continuous and inseparable. Utilization review should not, as it is under standard telephone UR programs, be characterized by angry, antagonistic, distant telephone exchanges between providers, patients and reviewers (Kertesz, 1988; Tarini, 1989). Rather, a highly managed system should be seamless and self-certifying, invisible to the patient, and fully integrated with the provider (Penzer, 1990).

Coordination is particularly important for treatment *sequencing*, matching service intensity with symptom acuity. Such sequencing is more important in mental health and substance abuse than in the standard medical/surgical PPO. In the standard PPO, a patient can mistakenly stumble into a network hospital and get full benefits. In a highly managed mental health and substance abuse PPO with an out-of-network option, someone who goes into one of the network facilities, but who does so out of sequence, will be considered out of compliance and will get the lower level benefits (Anderson, 1989).

Unlike a medical PPO, the highly managed "opt-out" mental health program will not even publish a directory of providers. Such directories encourage patients to contact a particular provider, out of sequence from the network's case management system, inhibiting cost-effective care (Kunnes, 1989).

Providers

The quality and cost of care are ultimately dependent on the providers of care and the contexts in which they provide it (Weiner, 1989). Practitioners and facilities should be specialized (Brazda, 1990) and sub-specialized to adequately meet the needs of patients. Without such specialization, it is difficult to match symptom acuity with service intensity and functional level with facilities (Herrington, 1989). An adolescent with an eating disorder, for example, who is not in immediate metabolic risk and expresses some vague suicidal ideation, can usually be treated in a very intensive outpatient or partial hospitalization program. This is possible as long as there is present in the treatment program, services for both adolescents and eating disorders (Lopez, 1989).

Sub-specialty mental health professionals are difficult to recruit, particularly by managed care programs. They are not sufficiently aware that a well managed, high quality provider network and managed care system can be very satisfying to work in, particularly if the benefit design emphasizes maximal coverage and quality. In such a scenario, psychiatrists and other mental health professionals can have the best of both possible worlds: their patient volume may be significantly increased; and because the benefits cover virtually all needed services, they can practice according to the basic tenets of their professions and clinical education.

Every employer has a different employee and dependent mix. The differences are in gender, age, socioeconomic status, educational level, utilization history, prevalence of diagnostic categories, geography, etc. The local mental health/substance abuse provider network must accommodate such variations. A group with significant numbers of teenage females, for example, is likely to require the availability of professionals who specialize in adolescent eating disorders. Another with a significant retiree population will require providers who specialize in geriatric depressive disorders. Failure to specialize and customize the provider network will result in an inability to match symptoms with service, increase the likelihood of recidivism and decrease quality.

Providers should be selected on the basis of their commitment to and experience in cost-effective, high-quality care. A good, well-managed system needs, like the Marines, only a few good ones. The quality of a provider network should not be measured by its size. Small, in a managed care context, is usually better. A small number of providers, geographically dispersed, carefully selected and continuously monitored, is a significant advantage over a large network that is likely to be more difficult to manage and to know well (Bradman, 1989). Careful credentialing means quality and cost-effectiveness are more likely to be assured from the beginning. A provider who fails to meet performance standards should be quickly and effectively educated. If it is not effective quickly, the provider should be extruded from the network. An "urge to purge" approach increases the likelihood of higher quality care and lower costs.

Cost Effectiveness

Quality of care is best determined more by what the patient does than what the patient feels. The quality of a managed mental health and substance abuse system must rest on sufficient improvement in the individual patient's *functional effectiveness* (Burda, 1989). The estimate of cost-effectiveness for the overall system must ultimately be based on similar, *measurable parameters* (Traska, 1989). From the insurer's perspective, the two most important ones are the functional improvement of all the patients treated; and the ability to show such improvement at a predictable and guaranteed claim level, at or below current claim costs. It may seem paradoxical to suggest that guarantees of lower claims expense can be a component of quality. However, effective managed care programs, particularly in the current context of very high costs and utilization, should have little difficulty in doing so. Any costs higher than eight dollars per covered *life* per *month* under a standard indemnity benefit design should, with a good managed care system, be reduced by 20 to 30%. This assumes significant disincentives for out-of-network utilization, i.e., 90% coverage for in-network and 60% for out-of-network. Inability to guarantee such a reduction suggests a poor management information system, particularly a poorly integrated management and treatment system. But the guarantees (Prospero, 1987) can be achieved only in the context of an appropriate benefit, management, and treatment system design.

Given the concern by insurance carriers and others about the magnitude of the money being wasted on mental health and substance abuse services, particularly on inpatient care, managed mental health has a great opportunity. The carriers also understand that care without quality is not cost effective; care that is not cost-effective is unlikely to be of quality. Cost-effective and quality care are not only measurable, simultaneous and synonymous, they are also synergistic. And this allows the system to do well by doing good, and to do good by doing well.

REFERENCES

Ad.: *EAP Digest,* 6:20, 1989.

Altshuler, K.: New Plan. *Psychiatric News, 34:*1,28, September 1, 1989.

Anderson, D. F.: Mental health PPOs. *Business & Health, 11:*34–35, 1989.

Bailey, N.C.: Does managed mental health care have a future? *Business & Health, 11:*26–28, 1989.

Bigelow, D.: Comparative costs and impacts of Canadian and American payment systems for mental health services. *Hospital & Community Psychiatry, 40:*805–807, 1989.

Bradman, L.H.: Contract directly for mental health care. *Business Insurance, 17:*49–50, 1989.

Bradman, L.H.: Direct contracts don't restrict patient choice. *Business Insurance, 17:*8–10, 1989.

Brazda, J.F.: Well-managed out-patient care seen best for substance abuse. *Managed Care Report, 3:*6, 1989.

Brazda, J.F.: In 1990: More managed care members. *Managed Care Report, 3:*1–4, 1990.

Brazda, J.F.: Indemnity plan costs rose 20.4%. *Managed Care Report, 3:*5, 1990.

Brightbill, T.: Mental health firms offer more care for less cost. *Contract Healthcare, 4:*9–11, 1988.

Bruce, M.L.: Psychiatric disorders and 15-month mortality. *American Journal of Public Health, 79:*727–730, 1989.

Bryant, M.: What can be done for troubled teens. *Business & Health, 11:*10–14, 1990.

Bukstein, O.G.: Comorbidity of substance abuse and other psychiatric disorders in adolescents. *American Journal of Psychiatry, 146:*1131–1139, 1989.

Burda, D.: Quality study uses patients' perceptions. *Modern Healthcare, 8:*4, 1989.

Bureau of Labor Statistics.: Employee benefits in medium and large firms. *Medical Benefits, 3:*1–2, 1989.

Cagney, T.: Managed care: A view of the future. *EAP Digest, 7:*47–52, 1989.

Cavaini, R.: Utilization review in mental health services. *Medical Interface, 3:*10–12, 1990.

Chasnoff, I.J.: Substance abuse commonly missed obstetric diagnoses. *Modern Healthcare, 8:*70, 1988.

Chodoff, P.: Effects of the new economic climate on psychotherapeutic practice. *American Journal of Psychiatry, 144:*1293–1297, 1987.

Coniaris, J.C.: Managed care. *Psychiatric News, 24:*19, August 18, 1989.

Connolly, J.: Psych care costs need trimming. *National Underwriter, 16:*18, 1988.

Cresson, F.: State mandates at issue. *GHAA News, 30:*19–22, 1989.

Darton, N.: Committed youth. *Newsweek, 115:*66–69, July 31, 1989.

DiBlase, D.: Bank blends HMO and indemnity plans. *Business Insurance, 17:*3,16, 1989.

Donkin, R.: The new mental health watch dogs. *Business & Health, 11:*16–18, 1989.

Droste, T.: Teens: Trading boarding schools for psych wards. *Hospitals, 41:*77–78, 1988.

Droste, T.: 1989. Employers want more substance abuse services. *Hospitals, 41:*24–30, 1989.

Duva, J.: Ask a benefit manager. *Business Insurance, 17:*4, 1989.

Erb, J.: Odds and ends. *The Wall Street Journal, 71:*B1, November 10, 1989.

Fauman, M.: Quality assurance monitoring in psychiatry. *American Journal of Psychiatry, 146:*1121–1129, 1989.

Fink, P.: APA issues position statement on adolescent hospitalization. *Psychiatric News, 24:*1,17, July 7, 1989.

Firshein, J.: Is U.S. health care ripe for reform. *Utilization Review, 18:*6–8, 1990.

Freudenheim, M.: More aid for addicts on the job. *The New York Times, 139:*D4, November 13, 1989.

Friedman, G.: Outcome study incorporates quality of life measures. *Health Week, 3:*4, August 28, 1989.

Fry, R.: The fiscal fitness of outpatient care. *Employee Benefit News, 19:*30–32, September 1989.

Gaver, K.D.: Balancing cost, quality of psych care. *Employee Benefit News, 19:*28–29, September 19, 1988.

Gelber, S.: Efficient MHSA care focuses on plan design. *Managed Care Outlook, 2:*1–3, October 27, 1989.

Gibson.: Private hospitals' share of mental services rises. *Modern Healthcare, 8:*14, 1989.

Gillig, P.M.: The psychiatric emergency service holding area. *American Journal of Psychiatry, 146:*369–371, 1989.

Glaser, T.: Outpatient residential treatment. *EAP Digest, 7:*68–70, 1989.

Goering, P.N.: What difference does case management make? *Hospital and Community Psychiatry, 39:*272–276, 1988.

Grumet, G.: Health care rationing through inconvenience. *The New England Journal of Medicine, 321:*607–609, 1989.

Hayashida, M.: Comparative effectiveness and cost of inpatient and out-patient detoxification. *The New England Journal of Medicine, 320:*358–364, 1989.

Hellerstein, D.J.: Outpatient group therapy for schizophrenic substance abusers. *American Journal of Psychiatry, 144:*1337–1339, 1987.

Herrington, B.S.: Cost containment measures will continue chokehold. *Psychiatric News, 24:*11–13, January 1, 1989.

Herrington, B.S.: Carving out mental health. *Psychiatric News, 24:*2, July 7, 1989.

Herrington, B.S.: JCAHO developing clinical indicators. *Psychiatric News, 24:*2, August 4, 1989.

Herrington, B.S.: Partial hospitalization under utilized. *Psychiatric News, 24:*1,19, September 15, 1989.

Herrington, B.S.: Outpatient managed care "inevitable". *Psychiatric News, 24:*16–17, November 3, 1989.

HIAA.: The price of state mandated benefits. *Medical Benefits, 6:*3, 1989.

Howard, L.S.: Benefit managers eye psych care costs. *National Underwriter, 16:*18–19, 1989.

Kenkel, P.J.: Utilization review takes toll on mental health units. *Modern Healthcare, 9:*42, 1990.

Kertesz, L.: Doctors sue over managed care program. *Business Insurance, 17:*44, 1988.

Kertesz, L.: McDonnell Douglas EAP trims costs. *Business Insurance, 18:*3, 1989.

Kim, H.: Tension typifies relationship between psychiatric providers and managed care. *Modern Healthcare, 7:*86–88, 1988.

Kim, H.: Psych providers reach out with message of comfort. *Modern Healthcare, 7:*50, 1988.

Kim, H.: Psychiatric facilities should listen to their market. *Modern Healthcare, 8:*42–44, 1989.

Klerman, G.: Efficiency of a brief psychological intervention. *Medical Care, 25:*1078–1087, 1987.

Klerman, G.: Treatment of alcoholism. *The New England Journal of Medicine, 320:*394–395, 1989.

Krantz, P.: Is your child hooked on drugs or alcohol. *Better Homes and Gardens, 62:*41–43, February 1990.

Kunnes, R.: Managed psych care. *Managed Care Outlook, 2:*7–8, December 22, 1989.

Levick, D.: Employers looking at ways to curb costs of mental health care. *The Hartford Courant, 153:*31, April 28, 1988.

Lopez, L.: Managing mental health. *GHAA News, 30:*6–9, September/October 1989.

Marsh and McLennan Companies.: A costly problem for corporate America. *Substance Abuse Issues, 1:*2–3, Winter 1990.

Moyer, D.: Unfazed by debt, Charter Medical sees gold in growth. *Health Week, 3:*11, December 18, 1989.

Melnick, G.: The growth and effects of hospital selective contracting. *Health Care Management Review, 14:*57–64, Summer 1989.

Millman, R.: Who will treat alcohol and drug abuse patients. *Hospital and Community Psychiatry, 40:*989, October 1989.

Mullen, P.: Study shows company health bills rose 18.6%. *Health Week, 3:*1,27, February 6, 1989.

Mullen, P.: Cigna buys firm to pare cost of mental care. *Health Week, 3:*14, February 6, 1989.

Nissen, T.: MCC targets mental health insurance. *Minneapolis/St. Paul City Business, 7:*11,17, January 15, 1990.

Pallarito, K.: Hospital ventures into deals with specialty providers. *Modern Healthcare, 8:*48, 1989.

Paris, E.: Sigmund Freud, meet Jean-Baptiste Say. *Forbes, 145:*148–152, February 19, 1990.

Penzer, W.N.: The realities of managed mental health care. *EAP Digest, 7:*35–43, 1990.

Pereira, J.: Firms cut drug treatment benefits. *Medical Benefits, 6:*5–6, 1989.

Prospero, A.R.: Selecting a case manager for psychiatric care. *Business & Health, 9:*32–33, 1987.

Prosser, P.E.: Mental health care needs careful review. *Business Insurance, 17:*8, 1989.

Rodin, B.: Managing psych benefits. *Managed Care Outlook, 2:*1–2, 1989.

Shadle, M.: The impact of HMO development in mental health and chemical dependency services. *Hospital & Community Psychiatry, 40:*1145–1151, 1989.

Smith, J.: Outpatients elude "pink cloud blues." *The Wall Street Journal, 71:*A23, October 4, 1989.

Tarini, P.: Managed care's hidden costs. *American Medical News, 33:*13–16, August 18, 1989.

Thomas, R.L.: Psych providers attack myths. *Managed Care Outlook, 3:*5–6, 1990.

Tigner, R.: Charter Hospital's aggressiveness sparks criticism. *The Business Journal,* (Phoenix) *9:*1, July 31, 1989.

Traska, M.: What one HMO company did. *GHAA News, 30:*18, September/October 1989.

Traska, M.: The case behind mental health carve outs. *GHAA News, 30:*14–17, September/October 1989.

Vibbert, S.: Utilization review: A report card. *Business & Health, 10:*37–44, 1990.

Weiner, R.: Managed mental health care issues and strategies. *Benefits Quarterly, 17:*21–31, 1989.

Wells, K.: The functioning and well being of depressed patients. *Journal of American Medical Association, 262:*914–917, 1989.

Wenzel, L.: Mental health options under HMOs. *Business & Health, 8:*30–33, 1988.

White, V.: Which benefit area of managed care plans is in need of the most improvement? *Medical Interface, 2:*6–7, 1990.

Whitted, G.: Psych case management will be altered. *Managed Care Outlook, 2:*1–3, 1989.

Winslow, R.: Spending to cut mental health·costs. *The Wall Street Journal, 7:*B1, December 13, 1989.

Wright, R.G.: Defining and measuring stabilization of patients. *American Journal of Psychiatry, 146:*10, 1989.

Chapter 7

MANAGED MENTAL HEALTH:
THE BUYER'S PERSPECTIVE

Joan Pearson

M any corporations are concerned about the mental health and substance abuse component of their employee health benefit plans,
primarily due to rising costs. They are considering, and a number have
already adopted, a managed mental health strategy. Some of these strategies are apparent to employees while others are not.

For many employers, mental health and substance abuse treatment
costs are the fastest rising segment of their medical plan costs. A recent
study (Alder 1989) reported that between 1988 and 1989 such costs, for
employers with over 1,000 employees, rose an average of 47%. Some
employers have reported that their 1989 costs are double that of 1988.

A comparative analysis (May 1988 through April 1989 compared with
the same period five years earlier) of the medical cost and utilization of
21 employer groups with over 200,000 employees (Information Management Bulletin, Fall 1989) concluded that:

> In contrast to the decline in inpatient medical/surgical utilization, the
> hospital admission rate for mental disorders increased by 37% and 47%
> for substance abuse during the study period. The average length of stay
> in hospitals increased for both conditions.

> The per person expenses for the treatment of mental disorders in-hospital
> increased by 132%, or an average annual rate of 18.2%. Expenses for
> treatment of substance abuse rose at an average annual rate of 21.7% per
> covered person in hospitals and 35.7% in specialized treatment facilities.

Experience shows that the rate of increase varies from one employer to
another. Those that have relatively low benefit limits (e.g., a $5,000
annual cap on inpatient treatment) experience much lower increases.
Companies with little or no special limits, however, are finding costs for
psychiatric and substance abuse treatment rising sharply. Rates also
differ by region. In May 1989, for example, room and board rates for

psychiatric hospital treatment in Philadelphia were reported at $613 per day; the Dallas rate was $293 (Open Minds, 1989).

Many factors have contributed to rising mental health and substance abuse costs:

- Supply-side factors: In part, cost escalations are supply driven. Between 1979 and 1986, inpatient psychiatric treatment facilities grew from 180 to 250 (Bassuk and Hilland 1987). By 1987, psychiatric hospitals numbered 324 (Hospitals, March 1988). Between 1986 and 1987 the number of psychiatric beds jumped 28%—from 24,008 to 30,633 (Hospitals, March 1988). To some degree, this growth reflects declining medical and surgical inpatient utilization, resulting hospital over-capacity and the conversion of such beds to psychiatric use.

- State mandates: Another impetus for these increases has arisen from state-mandated mental health and substance abuse coverage in insured health plans. States are increasingly requiring insurance companies to offer or provide this coverage in group plans.

- Ineffectiveness of traditional cost controls: The relative subjectivity of mental and substance abuse disorders has undermined traditional cost control programs, especially those that rely on diagnosis (e.g., utilization review programs). Diagnosis predicts lengths of stay for mental disorders so poorly that Medicare continues to pay for such inpatient care on a fee-for-service basis rather than on the basis of the diagnostic-related group reimbursement system.

- Juvenile court referrals: The juvenile court system increasingly uses treatment as a substitute for detention, especially for children who exhibit antisocial behavior. Some of these children are being warehoused because the schools, institutions for juvenile delinquents and parents are unable or unwilling to take responsibility for them.

- Societal acceptance of treatment: Finally, society has become more accepting of mental health and substance abuse treatment. This has resulted in higher demand.

Growing Concern About Quality

Employers are also increasingly concerned about the quality of care. There has been increasing publicity, for example, about adolescents who believe they have been harmed by lengthy, unnecessary hospital confinements, especially when they have been admitted involuntarily. Another quality of care issue is the high incidence of relapse after treatment for substance abuse. The Center for Applied Science (Donkin, 1989) found that about 50% of those treated for alcohol or drug abuse relapse within one year. Some corporations are seeking treatment programs that achieve higher success rates. The follow-up care provided after the completion of treatment is often a critical element in such success.

There is also increasing evidence that untreated mental health and substance abuse problems result in significantly higher utilization of other health care services and that successful treatment can reduce the use of those services. Early identification and prevention efforts—such as Employee Assistance Programs—are designed to encourage employees to get help before a problem becomes overwhelming.

Some of the quality problems associated with mental health and substance abuse treatment stem from faulty benefit plan designs. Often there are strong financial incentives for patients to seek inpatient treatment. Inpatient substance abuse treatment, for example, may be covered at 100% while outpatient treatment is covered at 50%, with a $1,500 annual benefit maximum. This type of plan design may cost the patient $2,500 for an outpatient program while inpatient treatment costs nothing. In addition, outpatient treatment coverage is usually inadequate for those with a chronic, debilitating psychiatric condition.

Significant Savings

When employers closely examine their mental health and substance abuse treatment experience, they often find that existing medical plan cost controls (e.g., utilization review) have little or no impact. Cost and utilization analyses indicate that significant reductions (e.g., 10% to 40%) can be achieved with managed mental health programs. In addition, there is considerable evidence that the quality of care provided can be significantly enhanced under managed mental health.

An analysis of inpatient utilization is a basic step in determining a company's need for a managed mental health program. This analysis focuses on inpatient stays and identifies opportunities to reduce those that are unnecessarily long as well as ways to purchase treatment more cost-effectively. Because the average mental health and substance abuse confinement has a length of stay about four times greater than in medicine or surgery, savings opportunities are more readily apparent. Further,

70% of mental health and substance abuse treatment costs are incurred for inpatient care, in comparison to 50% or less for medical/surgical. In addition, there is considerable variability between facilities with regard to the cost per day or per stay.

Managed mental health programs are also attractive because the disruption of existing provider relationships is minimal. A very small percentage of an employer's medical plan enrollees is in psychiatric treatment at any given time. An employed population generally has between five and six inpatient admissions per 1,000 covered lives. Of those who receive outpatient mental health treatment, about 80% complete it within 10 visits. For these reasons, very few are likely to have their treatment disrupted by a managed mental health program.

Deciding to Implement Managed Mental Health

The purchaser considers a number of things in deciding to implement a managed mental health program. Employers with fewer than 1,000 employees do not generally consider such a program. This is due in part to the small human resources staffs typically found in such companies. In addition, one of the savings opportunities in a managed mental health program is the negotiated discounts with selected providers. The limited utilization in a company with less than 1,000 employees generally makes such discounts less significant.

A major consideration is the cost experience of the medical benefits as a whole. An interest in managed mental health is usually spurred by a medical plan cost trend that is unacceptable to top management. In some cases, a company will have experienced relatively low plan cost increases for a number of years followed by a sharp increase. This sudden spike may lead to a thorough investigation of all cost saving opportunities. In other instances, a company's cost trend may have been unacceptable for some time despite numerous attempts to hold costs down. Another common factor in considering managed mental health is the belief that further cost shifting to employees is unacceptable and that other cost control alternatives must be sought.

Employers look at a number of indicators to determine if a managed mental health program would be cost effective. The most important of these is the utilization of inpatient days per 1,000 lives covered under the plan. If days per 1,000 exceed 100, there is a reasonable likelihood that some form of managed mental health program would be worthwhile.

Another key indicator is the point at which psychiatric and substance abuse benefit costs exceed 10% of total medical plan costs. Inpatient admissions per 1,000 covered lives (admissions per 1,000) generally are expected to be around six. Admissions in excess of 6 per 1,000 or an average length of stay over 21 are also indicators of the potential benefits of managed mental health. Finally, annual increases for mental health and substance abuse treatment that exceed 20% may suggest that costs are out of control.

MANAGED MENTAL HEALTH PROGRAM OPTIONS

A wide array of alternatives are available to employers interested in managing their mental health and substance abuse benefits. These are discussed below, beginning with the least restrictive from the perspective of access. Generally, savings will increase as access to treatment is both restricted and managed.

Implement Employee Assistance Programs

Many employers already have Employee Assistance Programs (EAPs) designed to provide assessment and referral services to employees and their dependents seeking help with personal problems. The primary purpose of an EAP is to match the employee's needs with an appropriate mental health professional. Increasingly, EAPs offer short-term counseling services that provide up to eight visits at no charge. About 70% of those who seek help from an EAP providing short-term counseling resolve their difficulties and do not require a referral for further assistance.

Many employers seek advice from their EAP staff about the reasons underlying treatment cost increases. In addition, EAP staff are being asked to participate in the design of the managed mental health program. Some companies ask their EAPs to manage the substance abuse treatment covered under the benefit plan. The EAP counselor assesses the need for and refers the patient for treatment, insures that the care is necessary and follows the patient after treatment is completed.

Revise Benefit Plan Design

Another avenue that must be explored in managing mental health and substance abuse treatment costs is the benefit plan design. Some plans may, for example, require an employee to pay more for outpatient than for inpatient services. This is a particular problem with substance abuse where outpatient care is appropriate for between 70% and 80% of those who need treatment. Although outpatient treatment is likely to be more effective and much less costly to the company, patients who have higher out-of-pocket costs for outpatient care are discouraged from using it. Because many outpatient treatment programs are offered in the evening, employees can continue to work. The employer avoids sick leave and replacement costs. If employees are required to pay more for outpatient treatment, however, they may select inpatient care instead and as a result, all these savings will be lost to the employer.

Another plan design issue has to do with the mental health professionals covered under the benefit plan. Some plans cover only the services of physicians. Psychologists and social workers are not included but there are a number of reasons they should be. First, physicians tend to be the costliest providers of mental health services. Although psychiatrists or other physicians must oversee the use of prescription drugs, patients who do not need to be medicated can often be treated more cost-effectively by other professionals whose fees are lower. The most common guideline is to cover those mental health professionals licensed to practice independently (which varies form state to state). All states license psychologists, generally those trained at the doctoral level. About half of the states also license social workers with masters degrees.

In addition to lower fees, psychologists and social workers—as non-physician practitioners—may be less intimidating to a potential client and, therefore, more likely to be sought out before a problem becomes acute.

Strengthen Existing Cost Controls

Another alternative is to strengthen existing utilization review and generic case management programs. This can be done through the use of stronger financial penalties for failures to notify the utilization review firm in a timely fashion that treatment is being provided. Another approach is to audit the effectiveness of existing cost controls and determine ways to strengthen them through such measures as early intervention or more aggressive discharge planning and aftercare.

Implement Specialty Case Management

In the event that the generic utilization review program is not sufficiently effective, a case management program can be implemented through a firm that specializes in managing mental health and substance abuse treatment. Specialty utilization review and case management offer the following advantages:

- Greater knowledge of alternative care available, particularly treatment "in between" traditional inpatient and outpatient services.
- Staff psychiatrist advisors who interact much more frequently with treating psychiatrists than typically found in generic utilization review programs.
- Higher use of extracontractual benefits, generally for intermediate care or additional outpatient visits.
- Strong promotion of discharge planning and aftercare.
- Emphasis on family participation in treatment, especially with children and adolescents. "Warehousing" children who create problems at home is less likely to be permitted.
- Psychiatric medications are closely monitored.
- Better coordination with the EAP.

Preferred Provider Network

The next level of managed mental health involves the use of a preferred provider network. A properly constructed network can make the most significant contribution to managing mental health and substance abuse treatment costs. One reason is the wide variability in provider charges for essentially the same treatment within the same community.

More important, unlike most medical and surgical care, there is little agreement among mental health practitioners on how to treat various disorders. Some use inpatient treatment extensively while others believe it should be used only sparingly. A managed mental health network seeks out the latter groups and the difference (in such utilization measures as inpatient days per 1,000) has been found to be statistically significant. Selecting mental health practitioners who believe in aggressive outpatient treatment is particularly important with psychiatrists. In most states, only psychiatrists can admit patients to hospitals. Because 70% of treatment costs are incurred in hospitals, psychiatrists exert the strongest influence on how the treatment dollar is spent.

Many employers using preferred provider networks allow employees to use non-network providers. At least a 30% coinsurance differential between in and out of network coverage is recommended to provide adequate steerage toward the network. In addition, employee out-of-pocket maximums are typically removed if non-network providers are used and benefit maximums are reduced.

Exclusive Provider Organization

A more restrictive managed mental health alternative is to limit coverage for mental health services to network providers only. Employees who choose non-network providers receive no reimbursement under the benefit plan.

Exclusive provider organizations (EPO) are becoming more common. As employers learn more about the costs of allowing employees open access to mental health treatment, they may opt for a totally managed mental health delivery system. Sometimes the EPO is limited to inpatient psychiatric and all substance abuse treatment. In these plans, open access to all covered outpatient mental health providers is permitted.

Quality may also be a major consideration in selecting an EPO. Some employers conclude that employees cannot find appropriate mental health care on their own. Primary care physicians are often unprepared to make a referral and are usually not asked for this type of advice. People are reluctant to discuss their mental health treatment needs and, in desperation, turn to the yellow pages or television advertisements for help. EPOs offer employees immediate, round-the-clock professional assistance and preclude the selection of a provider based on limited or poor information.

Customizing a Managed Mental Health Program

Some employers are choosing to carve out their mental health and substance abuse treatment benefits from the rest of the medical plan. Usually, the goal is not only to achieve significant cost savings in the indemnity medical plan but also to offer the same mental health benefits to HMO members. The reasons for removing psychiatric and substance abuse treatment from HMOs are discussed in more detail below.

There are a number of factors that shape a company's managed mental health program. Some are associated with the characteristics of the company itself and others are more specific to human resource concerns. One of these is centralization. Companies differ in the extent to which they are centralized. Some are involved in different businesses with decisions made at the local business unit level. Others have internal EAPs in some divisions and outside ones in others. To the degree possible, consistent administration of the managed mental health program is helpful.

The labor relations environment is another consideration. Many companies offer HMOs to their union employees and, as HMO members, they have been exposed to managed mental health programs. Other union members enroll in largely unmanaged indemnity plans. Union leaders tend to be more concerned about substance abuse than mental health problems because the former is more likely to involve employees (as compared to dependents). In addition, substance abuse problems are more likely to be associated with bad performance on the job. Union interest in substance abuse treatment gave birth to Employee Assistance Programs, many of which began as industrial alcoholism programs. They usually enjoy strong union support.

Companies generally introduce the managed mental health program first to salaried employees and then hope to negotiate the program later with the union. This represents a change in the historical pattern of negotiating benefit increases with the union first and then passing them along to the salaried work force. Labor union considerations may influence the level of coverage provided within the network. The visibility of the managed mental health program to union members may be affected as well. Typically, managed mental health programs require those wishing access to services to call an 800 number for a referral. A program designed for union members may allow dual access options, one of which may include a list of preferred providers who may be accessed directly.

A company's drug testing requirements also influence its managed mental health program. In some, employees who test positive for drugs must be treated in accordance with the applicable regulations. Testing requirements are likely to affect record-keeping, coverage and timeliness issues in substance abuse treatment for those who test positive compared to those employees who seek treatment voluntarily or due to a job performance problem. The managed mental health program must insure that both company and government regulatory requirements are met with any employees who test positive.

The EAP's involvement in the development of a managed mental health program can be critical to its success. This is especially true with an internal EAP. The role of EAPs varies with regard to their involvement with inpatient treatment. Assessment and referral only EAP programs are less likely to refer directly to inpatient treatment than are short-term counseling programs where there is a greater degree of clinical involvement with patients. In addition, EAPs are much more likely to work with employees than with their dependents and with substance abuse rather than mental health. EAP staff can be particularly effective in substance abuse treatment where the employee's job is in jeopardy.

In developing a managed mental health program, the EAP can help in evaluating local treatment facilities and mental health professionals. They know which facilities are being used by employees as well as their reputations. The EAP can also act as a monitor to help insure that employees receive appropriate and timely care. Access to care is often more of a problem than the availability of the coverage. A delay from when the need for treatment is identified to when the treatment begins can result in patients changing their minds and postponing needed care.

There has frequently been conflict between the managed mental health program and the EAP, with the EAP concerned about denials or delays in needed care. The managed mental health firm tends to be critical of the EAP because of what it may perceive to be a lack of concern about costs and reluctance to consider alternatives to inpatient care. It is not uncommon for the patient to get caught in the middle. A successful managed mental health program hinges, in part, on a coordinated effort between the managed mental health firm and the EAP.

Another factor that influences the development of a managed mental health program is the percentage of a client company's employees enrolled in HMOs. HMO mental health and substance abuse treatment is coming under increasing criticism, particularly from EAPs. The criticism most often heard does not focus on benefit limitations as much as on access barriers. These criticisms have recently attracted management attention with the advent of employee drug testing. The sensitivities associated with drug testing require timely evaluation and when appropriate, treatment of HMO enrollees who test positive. For these reasons, some employers have carved out mental health and substance abuse treatment from their medical plans as a separate benefit, some of which have separate claims paying operations.

Benefit plan design and administration are other human resources considerations. The degree to which the benefit design for psychiatric and substance abuse services must be consistent with the rest of the medical benefits will influence the parameters of the managed mental health program. Many indemnity plans, for example, use a common deductible followed by a coinsurance that applies up to an out-of-pocket maximum. One of the design features that can simplify a managed mental health program is the use of a copayment, which is a fixed cost (e.g., $15) per visit rather than a percentage of the cost of the visit. Copayments are much easier for a managed mental health network to administer.

In administering the plan, the managed mental health firm must interact with the client company's claims payment system. The degree to which the system is automated and the interface options available are likely to influence the effectiveness of the managed mental health program.

Corporate Decision Making

The decision making process about whether to implement a managed mental health program varies widely from one organization to another. Often the company has undertaken a broad-based review of its health care benefits and mental health is included in the review. In these situations, the question of whether to treat mental health and substance abuse differently from the rest of the medical plan is usually a key issue.

The number of people involved in the decision making process as well as the positions held by the participants are strongly influenced by the degree of centralized decision making in the company. Decentralized companies will typically have representatives from their major business units participating in the decision along with the corporate staff. These groups are typically composed of people with different perspectives and levels of insight into employee health benefits so the decision making process is likely to take longer than in a centralized company. Sometimes these committees are staffed by representatives of the business units who are charged with keeping their units informed and who help prepare recommendations to be acted upon by yet another group. Organization size also tends to be correlated with the number of people involved in decision making, although in highly centralized organizations, the decision makers may often number less than six.

The criteria used to select a managed mental health firm also vary between organizations. The overriding factor, however, is to select the firm best suited to the company's perception of its overriding needs. Sometimes, the interface with the existing claims paying system is a driving factor. In other situations, minimizing the likelihood of problems during implementation is most important. The company may also be drawn to particular aspects of a firm's approach to managing care. And there are situations where the personal chemistry between the company and the managed mental health firm's representatives is the deciding factor.

Implementing a Managed Mental Health Program

A managed mental health program is generally introduced along with other pay and benefits changes. Depending upon the complexity and restrictiveness of the managed mental health program, there may be a need to develop a detailed communication about it.

Communication with employees is one aspect of a managed mental health program that often does not get enough attention. Particularly in programs where employees are penalized for failing to use network providers and procedures, special attention must be paid to explaining the program in an understandable and thorough way. Communication is particularly challenging because the costliest treatment—inpatient psychiatric care—almost always occurs during a family crisis. Usually, families are unaware of the magnitude of a psychiatric problem until a crisis occurs. Insuring that the employee and the family understand how to access care, especially during an emergency, is critical to the success of the managed mental health program.

Another consideration in the implementation of a managed mental health program is the way in which exceptions are to be handled (i.e., decisions to override recommendations of the managed mental health firm). There needs to be a clear understanding between the company and the managed mental health firm about how these exceptions will be handled. To the degree possible, a minimum number of exceptions should be made and top management should be helped to understand the need for consistent handling of cases, using criteria of medical necessity. Insuring that a mutually satisfactory appeals process is available in the event of a dispute can also help.

Financial Arrangements

There are several ways to reimburse a managed mental health firm. Generally, administrative fees are paid on a capitated per employee per year basis. For network programs, the managed care firm may be willing to put some or all of its fees at risk, depending upon how the program performs. In addition, the employer may enter into a contract where savings beyond a targeted dollar amount are shared with the managed care firm. The financial arrangements can be more favorable with EPOs rather than PPOs in which out-of-network coverage is available.

To enter into either of these arrangements, the employer must have reasonably good cost and utilization data, particularly about inpatient treatment. Without good information, predicting expected costs, with and without managed care, is difficult. Outpatient data are typically less reliable but, depending upon the plan design, this may not be a significant problem. Obtaining acceptable data is usually difficult, especially when multiple claims payors are involved or when there has been a recent change in claims paying practices.

The Role of the Consultant

Consultants play a variety of roles in helping their client companies implement a managed mental health program. Perhaps their most important contribution is in helping companies understand the nature of the cost savings opportunities and the alternatives available for capitalizing on them. Quality of care issues must be considered as well, especially in light of the ongoing need for treatment for those with serious psychiatric disorders.

The consultant usually begins by educating the company about mental health and substance treatment, with special emphasis on how it differs from medical and surgical care. Another key role for consultants is to obtain and analyze cost and utilization data in order to identify areas where treatment may be inappropriate or too costly.

The consultant also identifies cost management alternatives that take the following factors into account:

- Locations and facilities where employees are currently being treated
- Benefit plan design
- Savings goals
- Acceptability of restricting access to providers
- Existing administration and design of health care cost control programs (e.g., utilization review)
- Labor relations
- Claims payment
- Employee Assistance Programs—staff perception and desired involvement

- Geographic location of employees
- Purchasing power or volume of inpatient utilization
- Availability of alternatives to inpatient care
- Employee communications
- Network availability and feasibility

The goal is to help the company fashion a managed mental health program consistent with its goals, culture and constraints. Bringing the benefits and the internal EAP staffs together to develop the program is an increasingly common element. Both have a vested interest in the outcome and, together, can usually develop a more effective program than either can alone.

Once the company has developed a preliminary program design, the consultant can assist in implementation. Often, a request for proposal must be written and distributed to prospective vendors. After the proposals are received, they are analyzed, summarized and presented. Proposal review is usually followed by selection of semi-finalists and semi-finalist presentations. Sometimes semi-finalist site visits are conducted prior to final selection. The consultant often has information about the managed mental health marketplace that can be important to the final selection.

Once a managed mental health program, including vendor selection, has been fully developed, there are implementation issues such as determining the claims interface, negotiating the contracts and preparing employee communications, all of which often require the consultant's involvement. Consultants can also help insure that the managed mental health program is no more complex, restrictive or expensive than is necessary. These programs can be costly and without a consultant, a company may purchase more managed mental health than it needs.

Post Implementation

Immediately after the program is implemented, the company will likely begin receiving complaints from three groups. Employees will complain if the care they feel has been promised is not provided or is restricted. Since entire families are in crisis during a psychiatric emergency, insensitive or inaccessible treatment will quickly be brought to the company's attention. The EAP also serves as a watchdog over the program and EAP criticisms as well as compliments are usually reliable indicators of the program's success. Finally, providers will express dissatisfaction if they believe the quality of care is being compromised, if the claims procedures are too cumbersome or if reimbursement is delayed.

Measuring the quantitative success of the managed care program depends, in large part, on the degree of confidence in the cost and utilization data prior to its inception. Financial success can be determined only if good pre and post data are available. Assuming that good data are available, the key indicators are:

- Days per 1,000 covered lives
- Cost per day
- Cost per stay
- Cost per employee and
- Mental health and substance abuse treatment costs as a percentage of total medical plan claims cost

The company should also monitor compliance with the program requirements (e.g., notification) as well as the incidence of employee and provider appeals of the managed mental health firm's decisions. Readmission rates are also useful in determining if patients are receiving proper aftercare.

Conclusion

Managed mental health and substance abuse treatment are still relatively new. Because they differ in some important ways from managing medical and surgical care, generic utilization review has not been effective in many instances. Managed mental health programs can result in significant savings but in order for them to do so, the client company must give a great deal of responsibility to the managed mental health firm. These firms exercise considerable influence over the care provided, from the selection of the providers to be used through the utilization review and quality assurance processes. There is generally a much higher degree of consensus on treatment protocols in general medicine than in mental health. In selecting a managed mental health firm, therefore, an employer is buying not just a manager of care but a particular approach to treatment for its employees. To be successful, efficient management, cost effectiveness and high quality must characterize whatever managed care firm and approach are selected.

REFERENCES

Alder, S.: Psychiatric costs are rising at large firms. *Business Insurance, 28,* 1990.

Are HMO's slamming the door on psych treatment? *Hospitals,* 50–54, 1988.

Bussuk, E. L., and Holland, S. K.: Accounting for high cost psychiatric care 38–41 *Business & Health,* 1989.

Donkin, R.: The revolving door of addiction. *Business & Health,* 16, 1989.

Rinaldo, D.: Employee health care data center: *Information Management Bulletin,* Utilization and Cost Patterns of the Eighties, Corporate Health Strategies, 2–3, 1989.

Chapter 8

INFORMATION SYSTEMS

Marvis J. Oehm

Significant advances in telephone and computer technologies have furthered the development of utilization management systems. The availability of toll-free telephone numbers, sophisticated automated call distribution, and the growing capacity and speed of computer systems (both local area network and mainframe) have permitted the rapid expansion of telephone-based utilization management.

In the 1970s and early 1980s, most utilization management programs operated by Professional Standards Review Organizations (PSROs) and Foundations for Medical Care (FMCs) were typically local or statewide (Gray and Field, 1989). Clinical staff visited hospitals to perform utilization review using open medical records. Telephone activities were largely limited to second opinions and limited preadmission review of the necessity for elective hospital admission. Computer systems supporting these programs were generally used for reporting and analysis and claims payment purposes. Staff collected data in the field or forms were mailed to a central entry or payment point and data were batch entered by support staff. Data bases were updated on an overnight or less frequent basis. Paper files and tickler systems were used to support the review process.

While state and local programs continue to exist, the primary growth has been in programs serving wider areas by telephone. The cost of on-site programs, as a result of the heavy investment required in clinical staff, and the desire of large employers to purchase uniform services nationwide, have fostered the development of telephone-based programs that offer the full range of basic hospital utilization management as well as specialized services. Specialized services include catastrophic or long-term case management, outpatient review, channeling to preferred providers (PPOs), management of mental health and chemical dependency utilization, and high-risk maternity screening.

The actual use of computers to support utilization management activities in the telephone environment is highly variable. Over the past four years, the author has had the opportunity to observe the operations of some 60 utilization management programs. Some continue to operate on a paper basis with batch data entry for reporting and analysis purposes. Others have successfully moved to a paperless environment, with all transactions completed on-line in real time. Many operate essentially duplicate paper and computer systems.

While the core of a highly effective utilization management program is the quality of its clinical staff and clinical decision making, effective review can be enhanced by good on-line computer support. While batch entry systems can offer good capabilities for internal management and quality control as well as reporting and analysis, these areas are not the focus of this chapter. Rather, it describes system features necessary for effective computer support of daily utilization management functions.

A computer system supporting utilization management has several objectives for day-to-day operations. These include greater efficiency in managing cases, accuracy and consistency of the review and better customer service. As review volume increases, manual files and management of active cases become increasingly cumbersome. Since more than one person may call regarding a case, location of paper files and creation of duplicate cases are common problems. If the utilization manager (UM) or clinical reviewer originating the case is busy, another staff member must either locate the paper file or take a message. In a fully computer-supported program, the case file is immediately available to both.

Creation of tickler files for manual follow-up reviews is relatively simple with a small volume of cases. As volume increases, the number of "missed" reviews increases in a manual system. A good computer system can generate daily case review schedules to permit more targeted use of clinical staff time. When the system does not fully support on-line utilization management, duplicate paper systems are maintained. Clinical staff use paper forms and data are entered, either by clinical or support staff, resulting in duplication of effort. In these programs, the computer system is essentially a back-up filing system used for reporting and analysis and last resort case look-ups.

A variety of computer system features can enhance accuracy. On-line eligibility files and cross-walks to review screens, for example, can minimize errors in provider and patient demographics and eligibility. On-line access to benefit plan requirements such as second opinion or ambulatory procedures can alert reviewers to targeted areas. On-line access to coding modules, clinical criteria and length of stay norms can help assure greater consistency among reviewers. Computer assignment of case sequence numbers, dates and times of notifications and reviews and generation of follow-up review dates help assure accuracy of information recorded for tracking the timeliness of the utilization management process. Rapid on-line data entry at the time a call is received can reduce the time spent in collecting demographic data, freeing the UM to focus on medical necessity issues. To the extent multiple UMs have access to case records on-line, the number of call-backs can be reduced.

In a few systems observed by the author, callers were placed "on hold" for extended periods of time (over two minutes) so that the UM could complete complex combinations of manual and computer look-ups. In other systems, a normal part of conversations with callers included "the computer is very slow, please bear with me," or "I am waiting for the computer to change screens." In these situations, providers who frequently access the utilization management program are inconvenienced. Instead of taking five minutes to complete a review, it may take twice as long, with much of the time spent "on hold" or waiting for the system to respond. In other systems observed, callers were placed on hold while paper files were located. Utilization managers unfamiliar with a case then had to attempt to review the case files while getting new information.

At best, all these behaviors, built around the lack of adequate computer support, give a caller the impression of lack of efficiency. At worst, they convey arrogance through an apparent disregard of the time wasted by the caller. They also place the UMs in a weak position because they must apologize for their inability to rapidly complete basic non-clinical functions.

In summary, a good computer system can improve overall efficiency and free clinical staff from clerical chores associated with review scheduling and filing. It can provide easy access to diagnosis and procedure codes, clinical criteria, patient and provider demographics, and benefit plan requirements, thereby enhancing accuracy and consistency. Finally, it can permit the UM to quickly establish an efficient and professional image with callers. It should be emphasized here, however, that a computer system is not a substitute for clinically appropriate utilization management. While this chapter deals specifically with information system requirements, the reader should remember that the computer information system can *enhance* clinical review, but should not drive it.

The remainder of this chapter deals with the characteristics of an effective computer information system from the user's point of view. In this context, users are broadly defined to include utilization management staff regularly accessing the system as well as callers who are engaging the services of the review program. Some of the features discussed are desirable but not absolutely essential—these are identified as such.

PRIMARY BARRIERS TO IMPLEMENTING A "PAPERLESS" ON-LINE SYSTEM

Management Resistance

A commitment from middle management is critical to the successful implementation of an on-line system. In some programs, middle and top management view data entry as essentially a clerical function that takes away from clinical review time. Key managers often distrust computers in general, feeling there is a loss of accuracy and control of information by giving up paper files. Lack of management computer literacy is another significant barrier to effective implementation.

Most health care professionals have used hard copy clinical records much of their working lives. Paper records and files are tangible and personal. They can be touched and kept at one's desk or workstation, ready for retrieval on demand (Kongstvedt, 1989). Paper files can be personalized with notes and "post-it" stickers, permitting staff to evolve individualized ways of storing and retrieving data and managing individual workflows. Paper files are familiar and reliable. Although files may be lost, information in them does not degrade or change.

Some middle managers express the belief that computer systems deprive professional staff of individual flexibility. They maintain that data are degraded and information put in cannot be accurately retrieved again. These attitudes result in improper training of staff as overall distrust of the system is communicated to clinical reviewers. Management resistance to the introduction of computer information systems in day-to-day operations is the principal limiting factor in 20% of the programs observed.

Staff Resistance

Clinical staff may bring "computerphobia" to the position or may pick it up from middle managers who are not computer literate. Comments such as "clinicians are not typists" and "data entry is a clerical function" reflect a basic lack of understanding of the potential value of an on-line system. Clinical staff, particularly physicians, often share many of the management views described above (Worthley and Disalvio, 1989).

A good on-line system should replace individualized methods of managing workflow, permitting staff and management to more easily track case review progress. Management ability to more easily track reviews may threaten less productive staff. Slack can be more easily introduced into a particular staff member's workflow in a paper system than in a good on-line system. Utilization managers who are accustomed to using individual clinical judgment when making review decisions may feel the computer will force "cookbook" decisions. Computerized protocols and decision trees built into some systems force even the experienced UM to go through all the screens prior to making a review decision.

Typing skills, particularly for professional women, have traditionally been viewed as less than desirable, stereotyping women as clerks and secretaries. In a computer world, the ability to use a keyboard should eventually become as routine as using a pen or pencil. The computer system should be viewed as a tool, with more emphasis placed on *what* is entered than on *how* it is done. Note entry is not medical transcription and should not be viewed as such. Staff resistance can be minimized by line managers who are committed to computer system implementation.

Cost

In more than half the programs observed, the principal barrier to developing and implementing an effective system was cost. These programs are heavily invested in existing information systems, many of which were originally intended for claims payment. As such organizations developed utilization management capabilities, these activities were supported by paper systems or modules added on to the claims system. In some organizations, systems developed specifically for utilization management were quickly overloaded by rapid growth and expansion of service lines.

For all these programs, cost considerations include programming time as well as capital resources. In carrier-based programs, there are competing demands for programming time between claims and utilization management. As programming priorities are set, utilization management needs are frequently assigned a lower overall priority. In freestanding programs, capital and programming costs of system upgrades to accommodate growth are the principal limiting factors.

Rapid Response and Infrequent Down Time

If management, staff and cost barriers can be surmounted and a commitment made to implement an on-line system, its effective implementation will require surmounting one further barrier: actual speed and reliability. The most comprehensive, well designed system simply will not be properly used unless it is fast enough to accommodate on-line transactions and reliable enough to permit easy retrieval of all the information entered.

Response time is defined as the time, in seconds, it takes to complete a transaction. Down time is defined as the time(s) the system is not available and cannot be accessed by the users. Ideally, response time should accommodate real time entry and transaction times of 10–20 seconds. System down times should be infrequent events and, except for evening hours, should be related to significant power failures or similar problems. Frequent system-caused down time will result in the need to maintain a duplicate paper system. Slow response with repeated "system busy" messages and frequent down time are the two principal reasons duplicate paper systems are maintained.

From the point of view of the user in a telephone-based program (either the staff member or the caller), slow response time and down time have similar consequences. If response time is slow, in order not to inconvenience callers by requiring them to hold on the line until the computer responds, reviewers will use a paper form and enter the data later. If the system is down frequently, the UM will maintain paper backups so basic work can proceed without the system. When paper forms are used, data are generally batch entered into the system. If UMs do this, there is generally good correspondence between the data from the paper form and that entered into the system. If clerical or other support staff perform batch entry, clinical staff must often re-write notes to assure accurate entry. If paper backup is required on a weekly or more frequent basis, the primary system will be a manual or paper-based system.

In 70% of the programs observed, utilization management was supposed to be done on-line. However, only 5% of the programs had successfully eliminated duplicate paper systems, largely because of one or more of the factors listed above. The most common limiting reasons were poor system speed and reliability.

CHARACTERISTICS OF AN EFFECTIVE SYSTEM

Maximum user friendliness is required if clinical staff are expected to fully utilize the system. Identification of specific user requirements is the result of a combination of observations of successful systems and user problems in less successful ones.

The operational requirements of a highly effective utilization information system (from the user point of view) are summarized below. They focus on those aspects of utilization management, which, if properly implemented, will minimize clerical chores and permit clinical staff to devote maximum time to clinical review. Following the summary table, each characteristic is discussed in more detail.

System Characteristic	Essential	Desirable
System Speed and Reliability		
Permits on-line, real time transactions and file updates	x	
Is accessible more than 98% of the time during operating hours	x	
Demographic and Provider Data		
On-line facility files with crosswalks to review screens	x	
On-line clinician files with crosswalks to review screens		x
On-line lists of preferred providers with geographic or zip code search capability	x	
On-line lists of second opinion clinicians with specialty and geographic search capability	x	
On-line eligibility files with crosswalks to review screens		x
General Review Requirements		
On-line summaries of benefit plan review requirements		x
On-line clinical criteria with look-up capacity		x

On-line automated coding of diagnoses and procedures	x	
Space to retain admitting diagnosis, up to 5 discharge diagnoses and up to 5 procedures	x	
System flags for ambulatory procedures, second opinion procedures, questionable admitting diagnoses, case management diagnoses, readmissions	x	
Automated link to claims (in carrier based systems)		x
Case Review Support		
System automatically assigns case numbers	x	
System automatically records date, time, operator ID for transactions	x	
System generates follow-up review dates with flags for weekends and holidays and reviewer override capability	x	
System generates tickler files or case review scheduling reports	x	
Case summary screen, automatically updated as each review is completed	x	
Patient name search capacity	x	
Patient or employee social security number search capacity	x	
Case or certification number search capacity		x
Access to prior admissions and/or prior treatment files	x	
Capacity to complete a review based on a conversational flow of data	x	
Capacity to complete review, including pend capability, when some demographic data are lacking	x	
Capacity to suspend a record and go to another record without losing partial data entry	x	
Free text screens with sufficient page adding capacity for extensive clinical notes required for long-term or complex cases	x	
On-line length of stay norms with clinical reviewer override capability	x	
Forward and backward paging in an inquiry mode	x	
Capacity to add clinical information without creating a new review or requiring assignment of additional days to existing certifications	x	

Letter and certification generation capability	x

System Speed and Reliability

As discussed above, lack of speed and reliable access are the most common problems observed. In addition to the specific problems already discussed, in some systems, files are updated overnight. This means new cases or new information on existing cases will not be accessible until the next business day. As a result, staff may create duplicate records or duplicate updates for the same patient. This not only wastes staff time but can cause confusion among patients and providers if different UMs authorize different numbers of days or services for the same case.

In the worst situation observed, providers recognized the lag in the system and the UM's inability to effectively track current cases. Since the UMs did not follow their own cases and consistency could not be monitored through the system, providers would call around to different staff to get an answer they liked. To counter this practice, UMs would try to keep callers on the line, often "on hold" for long periods in an attempt to complete the review through a complex combination of computer and manual look-ups.

Rapid access to complete case files is particularly important in mental health and chemical dependency. In most of these programs, UMs follow their own cases so they have basic familiarity with the patient. Since the UMs frequently deal with the same providers, lack of ready access to complete case information puts them at an immediate disadvantage. The provider probably has the complete record in hand and must wait for the reviewer/case manager to locate a paper file. Immediately, the UM is in an apologetic mode, setting a different tone for the conversation.

Maintenance of parallel paper systems is the most common response to inadequate computer speed and reliability. In the worst case observed, the UMs would write all the information on paper forms (using the computer only for inquiry). After review was complete, they would carefully and painstakingly condense and summarize the information, making extensive use of various colored inks, so that clerical staff could enter the data on a batch basis.

In another program observed, the UMs recopied the clinical information and then entered it themselves into the system as time was available.

This is the most common solution in mental health and chemical dependency programs because of the complexity and detail of clinical data required for effective review. In the best case observed, the UMs maintained only a telephone log, checking off the type of call using a scratch pad, and the day's review schedule. Most of them were able to complete entry of clinical notes on-line during the conversation or within several minutes after it.

Demographic and Provider Data

In half of the programs observed, the greatest amount of time is spent on collecting and recording demographic data on employees, patients, hospitals and clinicians. Even in programs that serve defined areas with a limited number of hospitals, the same hospital data are collected for each new case. In some programs, calls are initially answered by support staff who take demographic information and direct callers to other sources if appropriate. If support staff perform initial intake in a manual program, the paper is passed to a UM for call back and follow-up. In some computerized programs, support staff are able to transfer the call to a UM who is able to retrieve the case through the computer and begin the clinical work. In other programs, calls are automatically distributed to an available UM who takes the demographic data and initiates the clinical review.

Regardless of the program configuration, effective on-line support can minimize staff time devoted to collection of basic demographic data. At a minimum, hospital or other facility files should be accessible on-line. The number of hospitals and free-standing facilities is reasonably manageable. Various directories such as the American Hospital Association Guide provide basic demographic data required to establish the file. Staff should be able to search by facility name, state and city to rapidly locate it. Facility name, address, telephone number and tax number should be brought automatically to the review screen when the correct facility is located. Good facility files can also store data on negotiated prices that can be used for case management purposes. Preferred provider status and information on special services offered can also be maintained.

In the best systems observed, provider files are also on-line. These files are often based on claims files or on historical review files. They generally contain name, address, telephone, and specialty. Staff can search for them by specialty, city and zip code. When the appropriate provider is located, these data are automatically brought into the review screen. For those organizations offering second opinion or clinical consultation services, this type of provider file is essential. Information on the quality of second opinion decisions or clinical consultations should be maintained and updated regularly. This permits staff to locate quickly quality providers when referrals are required.

In the ideal system, eligibility files are accessible on-line. Most utilization management program staff, including those with insurance carriers do not actually verify coverage and eligibility. Access to these files can, however, prevent significant misunderstandings. If there are any questions concerning eligibility (e.g., the employee is not listed) or coverage (e.g., a planned service may not be covered), the UM can refer the caller to claims or benefits management staff.

The most frequent problem with obtaining on-line access to eligibility files is that employers do not often have accurate files or positive enrollment. In the absence of data, utilization management programs must record employee and patient information on each case. When employees access clinical services intermittently, demographic data from prior records should be transferrable to the new case, minimizing some duplication of effort. When eligibility files can be obtained, demographic data should be automatically brought to the review screen.

Benefit Plan Summaries

The need for on-line summaries of benefit plans and general information about a company may vary with the overall configuration of staffing within the utilization management organization. Those with large employer contracts may have UM staff dedicated to particular employers. In these situations, on-line benefits information is not necessary. Other programs may deal with a variety of smaller employers with differing plan requirements and corporate cultures. Utilization managers may be involved with a number of different plans. In these situations, on-line benefits information is essential. Whether maintained on-line or in hard copy, this information should be centrally updated. Individual staff should not be responsible for compiling their own updates.

Clinical Criteria

There are a variety of opinions about the need for on-line access to clinical criteria. In a few of the programs observed, UM staff *must* respond to a series of clinical decision trees in order to reach a review decision. These same programs have mandatory referrals that cannot be overridden. Updates to these types of programs are time-consuming and expensive. In other programs, criteria can be accessed in an inquiry mode and are used for reference purposes. The ease of updating depends on the type of system and its general flexibility. In the majority of programs observed, clinical criteria are available in hard copy, with varying degrees of accessibility to staff. Accessibility ranges from staff not being able to locate a copy of the criteria but knowing it exists "somewhere," to well-thumbed criteria sets at each desk.

The principal problem with on-line decision trees is that they cover common diagnoses and procedures with which UMs should be very familiar. Over time, their use appears to result in boredom and a rote approach to the utilization management process. Unusual cases are difficult to accommodate and usually require a physician referral.

In mental health and chemical dependency programs, decision-tree criteria are difficult to implement because the UM must take into account a wide variety of factors in evaluating care requirements. On-line criteria with look-up capability or hard copy criteria for each staff member are the most reasonable solutions in these programs.

Automated Coding and Space

In the best systems observed, the UM can enter English language diagnoses or procedures and the system will automatically assign the codes for reporting purposes. Automated coding promotes consistency and reduces staff time devoted to coding functions. The more complex the coding requirements, the more important this feature is to make effective use of clinical time.

In a third of the systems observed, limited space to retain diagnoses required the admitting diagnosis to be replaced with updated information. By losing this information, management is unable to evaluate how initial reviews are being handled. Complex or long-term cases may have several diagnoses and procedures. For full tracking and analysis, the system should capture at least five diagnoses and procedures.

System Flags

Automatic system flags are one of the most useful and underused features of an on-line system. Flags can alert the UM to potential problem areas that may require access to criteria or possible referral to a clinical advisor. Flags can alert the UM to probe carefully when performing initial review. Most frequently, these flags are limited to second opinion procedures, ambulatory procedures, and diagnoses with case management potential. A variety of other flags are extremely useful, particularly in specialized utilization management programs.

"Problem" provider flags can be extremely helpful. In mature programs with track records for specific providers, these flags can alert the UM to special case review requirements such as requesting clinical records prior to continuing certifications.

For chemical dependency and mental health programs, flags denoting multiple admissions are extremely helpful. They alert the UM to a prior history which, if assessed, may help identify the need for alternative treatment planning. In the best system observed, a flag denoted the number of admissions for a particular patient.

Automated Claims Link

This feature is desirable in carrier-based programs. Information from the review screens should be automatically transferred to the claims system to permit payment to be made on the basis of correct review information. Ideally, most claims could be adjudicated through the system and not require manual assessment of the review documentation.

System-Assigned and Generated Data

The system should automatically assign the case numbers. A few "computerized" programs still require manual assignment of case numbers based on lists distributed each morning.

Accurate tracking of review timeliness requires that the system record dates, times and operator ID on all transactions. If notification penalties are applied, system generation of first call dates is critical for fair application of penalties. Dates of all review entries should be system generated. In the worst case observed, none of the dates could be used to evaluate timeliness of notification or review because they were "soft" dates. Staff frequently backdated reviews or split one review into two dates because "the computer would not accept more than X days on one review." In this case, it was not possible to accurately track the utilization management process. Staff were unable to accurately schedule follow-up reviews because none of the prior dates were accurate. In most programs observed, conduct of timely follow-up reviews was the weakest program component. Few programs accomplished more than 50% of the scheduled reviews on time. A large part of the problem was manual assignment of follow-up dates and manual tickler files.

When manually determined, review dates often fall on holidays or weekends and, as a result, are delayed until the following week. Staff may deliberately build in slack when manually assigning such dates to avoid heavy incoming call days. The best alternative is for the system to generate the follow-up date based on the days initially assigned. An override field should be provided so the UM can adjust the date if it falls on a holiday or clinical circumstances warrant a longer review interval. By maintaining both target and actual follow-up dates, the timeliness of follow-up reviews can be realistically assessed.

A case summary screen is an extremely useful feature found in only a few systems observed. With this feature, date of the last review, days assigned and next scheduled review date are transferred to a summary screen that includes the patient demographic data, diagnoses, procedures and length of stay to date. This type of screen is useful to perform a quick status check in response to an inquiry call.

Search Capabilities

The single most useful search function is on patient name. In the best systems, name searches can be performed for similar sounding names to accommodate misspellings. Frequently, callers (especially treating clinicians) will not have the case number or even the patient's social security number. On a name search, hospital name and admission date should be brought up in addition to the patient name. Patient name, hospital name and hospital admission date are the most common elements immediately available to most callers. If there are two or more patients with these three elements in common, birth date or social security number can be used to identify the patient. Many systems rely on the social security number as the primary search mode. Unfortunately, treating clinicians calling back may not have this information. This capability is most useful for facility contacts.

The case or certification number is the least useful from the callers' point of view. Some systems can only retrieve a case with its own unique number. Patients and employees may have recorded the number and many hospitals routinely record these number but clinicians often do not.

Access to Prior Treatment

While on-line storage may be limited, the UMs knowledge of prior admissions can help focus review in a current case. In mental health and chemical dependency programs such information is essential. If there has been a previous pattern of annual admissions for drug or alcohol dependency to the same or similar facilities, the UM may wish to explore other treatment options, including residential or structured outpatient programs.

Easy access to prior records can place the UM in a position of strength relative to the provider. The UM is able to knowledgeably discuss the patient's history, rather than relying solely on the provider for such information.

Conversational Data Flow

The majority of systems observed do not permit a normal conversational flow. In only one system was there an initial system prompt for the caller's name. In the vast majority of systems, this is the last item requested.

Utilization management is a service. When patients are actually accessing the system, they frequently do so in times of crisis, requiring some sensitivity on the part of the utilization management program. Most programs fall short in this area, often as the result of system demands for information in a particular order before moving to the next element.

Practitioners or patients calling to report an admission are frequently "cut off" by demands for detailed demographic information before they can complete a sentence. When support staff take initial calls and input demographic information, an impersonal approach during the first call may be necessary. When calls are automatically distributed to the UM, however, the system should permit movement between screens to follow normal conversational flow. In these situations, the only required element to initiate review should be the employee ID number, usually the social security number. In the best systems, the basic demographic information can be obtained at any time during the conversation.

Pend and Suspend Capability

The ability to pend or suspend cases can be a chronic problem in a utilization management program, resulting in large numbers of incomplete cases. Staff fail to obtain complete data and pend or suspend cases that are never completed. To guard against these problems, many systems have built in edits that prevent movement out of a screen or record prior to completion of required demographic fields. While such edits are well-intentioned, they can have unexpected results. In the worst case observed, callers were advised to call back when they had the telephone number of the facility. No information was recorded on these calls.

Managed properly, however, these features can enhance customer service and facilitate efficient review. Staff responding to telephone calls need to be able to move between records without losing data previously entered. If good provider files are maintained, delays in initiating a case should not depend on the caller's ability to provide all the demographic information. The principal method to guard against misuse of this function is a daily listing of these cases, with completion required by the end of the business day.

Free Text

The lack of free text for clinical notes is one of the most common problems in the on-line systems observed. In the worst case observed, limited space resulted in prior notes being overwritten so that no details on prior reviews were available. Some reviewers printed out notes before overwriting, others did not. In many other systems, notes had to be condensed to fit into available space. Condensing notes frequently consumed more staff time than would have been spent entering the detailed notes.

In mental health and chemical dependency programs, virtually unlimited free text is essential to track progress. These screens should be viewed as progress notes and not as minimal discharge summaries. Clinical notes provide the best basis on which to judge the quality of clinical decision-making. A number of systems observed rely on codes from criteria sets to support decisions. When these coding schemes are analyzed, the results show that individual staff tend to routinely use a limited set of codes, regardless of the categories of cases reviewed. Reliance on coded compliance with criteria is no substitute for proper clinical notes.

On-Line Length of Stay Norms

Based on the diagnosis and procedures entered, the system should generate a recommended length of stay. The system should also permit the UM to override this with fewer or more days, based on all the case factors. On-line reference points can help assure consistency of review. Over time, UM decisions should be compared against these reference points to assess overall performance.

Lack of on-line norms can have unusual results that present a poor image to the provider community. In one program observed, for the same patient and the same treatment, different UMs approved five different lengths of stay, ranging from one to five days. In another program, days approved over a six month period were compared with on-line length of stay norms for each UM. The range was a total of 168 days *less than the norm* to 1,700 days *more than the norm*. This level of variation should be unacceptable. These types of analyses are not possible without computerized review.

For mental health and chemical dependency programs, differences among UMs can be dramatic. Many programs have review intervals of seven days. Some have limits before going to a clinician advisor, others do not. In one program observed, some UMs consistently approved the entire number of days originally requested. Others consistently approved half the projected stay and successfully diverted cases to alternative programs.

Updating Clinical Information

Multiple calls may be required to obtain clinical information necessary to support approval of admission or length of stay. Edits in some systems automatically generate a new review with a requirement to assign days each time notes are updated. This results in an inaccurate number of days approved. Staff should be able to access a case to update clinical information without any additional systems requirements to exit.

Paging and Letter Generation

To the extent a program requires letters of certification forms, these should be automatically generated by the system.

Forward and backward paging is a useful feature, frequently overlooked in even the best systems. The more extensive the case notes, the more important this feature. Mental health and chemical dependency and case management programs cannot function well without it.

Training Needs

Effective training programs can be formal or informal, depending on how well existing staff and line management have adapted to the system and how easy it is to use. The principal training requirement is sensitivity to possible staff reluctance to give up paper systems. System reliability must be demonstrable.

Training should not focus on typing skills, particularly in free text entry. Rather, it should emphasize those features of the system that will free clinical staff from clerical chores and allow them to focus on utilization management rather than tracking functions. Materials should be simple and easy to follow. They should start with basics on how to access the system.

Minimum Case-Specific Data Collection Requirements

The following is a listing of the minimum data elements required for effective utilization management. All should be available on-line.

Demographic Data

Employer ID number
Employee, enrollee or subscriber ID number, name, address, relation to patient, telephone number (work and home)
Patient ID number, name, address, relation to employee, enrollee or subscriber, telephone number (work and home)
Patient age and sex
Hospital (facility) name, address, telephone, hospital (facility) number
Treating clinician name, address, telephone number
Second opinion or other clinician referral name, address, telephone number

Case Review Tracking Data

Case number
Operator ID number—each transaction
Notification date and time
Initial review date and time

Source of notification (patient, employee, enrollee or subscriber, facility, clinician)

Admission date (planned or actual)

Type of admission (emergency, urgent, elective)

Dates of scheduled follow-up reviews (system generated)

Dates of actual follow-up reviews (system-entered at the time of actual transactions)

Verified discharge date

Clinical Data

Admission diagnosis

Up to five additional diagnoses

Up to five procedures

Dates for up to five procedures

Patient disposition or discharge status

Case management status

Clinical case notes, including clinician advisor notes

Days requested and initial length of stay assignment (for comparison with length of stay norms)

Days requested and days assigned, each follow-up review

Second opinion indicators, including specification of waived, required, concurring or non-concurring

Results of any clinical referral or evaluation

Date(s) of referrals to clinician advisors

Packaged Programs Versus Internal Design

The most effective systems observed were internally developed and maintained. Packaged systems are most frequently operated independently of any basic internal systems. In the worst case observed, clinical reviewers moved between three computer terminals to access three different systems to complete a single review.

Packaged systems are most economical if they can be used without modification and there are no requirements to interface with existing systems. If there are interface requirements, the cost of programming the interfaces can be as expensive as developing a unique internal system. Buyers should carefully assess the flexibility of packaged systems to accommodate changes and increases in volume (Lackey, 1989). The costs of internal versus external maintenance and modifications should also be carefully assessed. While a packaged program may be useful in the early stages of implementation, it may not have the flexibility to accommodate rapid growth or expansion of service lines.

General Recommendations

System design, modification and implementation should be approached from the users' point of view, broadly defined to include staff and callers. Speed, reliability and flexibility should be the primary considerations. If these elements cannot be achieved, management should accept the inevitability of a paper system and accommodate staffing and basic program design, at least temporarily, to a paper system with batch data entry.

Under these conditions, rapid growth cannot be easily accommodated without overstaffing to compensate for the inefficiencies. In some programs observed, staffing was based on a "presumed" rather than actual computer system capabilities, with resulting significant delays in the overall utilization management process.

To the extent duplicate paper systems create inefficiencies and higher costs, organizations will not be harmed if the utilization management process remains effective and prices do not increase to reflect the inefficiency. Customer service implications should also be carefully assessed. Long hold times, frequent delays and retrospective reviews all have potential customer service implications.

Programmers and analysts must interact with UMs to determine actual system requirements. Programming staff should spend substantial time sitting with UMs to determine how the system is being used and how it can be improved. The worst example of distance between staff was observed in a program with a very elaborate computer system, capable of collecting hundreds of data elements. After a demonstration of the system and a review of its capabilities, the author joined the UM staff. Utilization managers were operating a paper system and several key system features lauded in the demonstration had never been implemented.

An elaborate system is not a substitute for effective utilization management, but a simple fast and reliable system can free UM staff from clerical chores and enhance the process.

REFERENCES

Gray, B.H., and Field, M.J. (Eds.): *Controlling Costs and Changing Patient Care? The Role of Utilization Management.* Institute of Medicine, Washington, D.C., National Academy Press, 1989.

Kongstvedt, P. (Ed.): *The Managed Health Care Handbook.* Rockville, Maryland, Aspen, 1989.

Lackey, J.V.: Claims and benefits administration. In Kongstvedt, P. (Ed.): *The Managed Health Care Handbook.* Rockville, Maryland, Aspen, 1989.

Worthley, J.A., and Disalvio, P.S.: *Managing Computers in Health Care.* Ann Arbor, University of Michigan Press, 1989.

Chapter 9

EVALUATION OF
MANAGED MENTAL HEALTH PROGRAMS

Joseph Smith and Gary L. Gaumer

The rapid development of managed care has outpaced attempts to carefully examine its results. Hundreds of different managed care companies are now offering programs to employers, programs that often differ from each other. At the same time, there is little empirical evidence that can be used to compare programs or to assess which work and which do not. The challenge is to develop workable approaches to evaluate managed care programs, approaches that provide information on the effects of managed care and on why and how the effects occur. This would allow the decisions that will ultimately shape managed care programs to be made with less reliance on anecdotes, hearsay, and vested interests.

The evaluation of managed mental health programs is particularly difficult. One important example is quality of care. Most quality assessment efforts have focused on the quality of inpatient care and have relied on the review of inpatient records. To evaluate the quality implications of a managed mental health program, however, one major question is whether or not access to inpatient services is inappropriately denied. To answer such a question, it is necessary to review outpatient records or collect other data on patients who have not been admitted to inpatient care. It is generally more difficult to get access to outpatient records, and the quality of documentation makes quality assessment difficult.

Another particularly difficult problem in the evaluation of managed mental health programs is that managed care is not a single entity. Managed care companies offer a wide variety of different products, and purchasers can choose from among them. Further, purchasers may choose to integrate the managed mental program into a particular benefit plan with its own limits, cost sharing, provider arrangements and other provisions. And finally, each individual managed mental health program is likely to be changing over time with regard to utilization review screens, case management staff and service alternatives. All this diversity makes it difficult to determine how to replicate successful outcomes and avoid failures.

This chapter is concerned with the problem of determining the effects caused by the implementation of or changes in a managed mental health program. Since such programs must be implemented in the real world, for clients with widely varying demands, it is not possible to proceed as would be the case with evaluating a clinical trial where there are clearly defined treatments as well as carefully matched control and treatment groups. Rather, the challenge is evaluating operational programs. As such, the basic questions that must be answered are:

- What happened?
- Why did it happen?
- What is the practical importance of what happened?

The question of what happened is far less trivial than it may appear. Managed mental health programs are complex, evolve over time, have staff changes and undergo varying degrees of transition and turbulence. This is far from an ideal experimental situation. In such an environment, it can be difficult to clearly define the treatment or when it became effective. This is in addition to the problem of measuring the outcome and comparing it to what it would have been without the treatment.

More complex than the question of what happened is why it happened. In mental health, there are a large number of factors that can make simple measures of outcome fluctuate wildly even with no "treatment" effect. Technological change, various pressures on established practice patterns, and reimbursement reform are among the more important ones. Further, in the period during which a managed mental health program is being implemented, the provider community may well be changing behavior in order to adapt, and people may be changing the way they select health benefit plans in response to changing options.

Assessing outcome is particularly difficult in mental health. The level of care required by any particular individual is a function of both trait and state characteristics. Trait characteristics include basic demographics— age, gender, diagnosis, and the individual's support system. These are relatively stable over time and measurements taken at discrete intervals can be applied for the entire period. State characteristics, on the other hand, can change from one day to the next and greatly affect the level of services required. These characteristics include items such as level of hallucination, family crises, and patient compliance with treatment protocols.

Another important issue to address is the question of the extent to which any particular characteristics of the population studied contributed to the effectiveness of the managed care intervention. The effectiveness of a managed mental health program in an underserved rural area, for example, is likely to differ from what would be true in a competitive environment where practitioners and facilities do not have a sufficient number of patients. The challenge here is to develop an evaluation strategy that enables the effects of the managed care program to be isolated from outcome differences caused by variations in patient and environmental factors.

The third basic question, dealing with practical significance, is an important one, too often overlooked. Evaluation results should serve the intended purpose. If the evaluation question concerns the cost effectiveness of a managed mental health program, it is not sufficient to determine just that managed care will reduce the cost of benefits. The administrative costs of the managed care program are also important. Similarly, if a purchaser of a managed mental health program has a young, mostly single employee population, evaluating a program for an older, married population does not meet the need. Another factor important to whether evaluation results have some practical use is the question of replicability. If a program is conducted haphazardly, without uniform training of participants and consistent or accurate collection of data, then the treatment cannot be recreated, and the results of the evaluation will have no practical value.

TARGETING THE EVALUATION

The single most important step in any evaluation is to define clearly the interventions that are being evaluated and to determine the correct evaluation questions.

Defining the Intervention

The intervention or treatment is the entity or system that is to be evaluated. For some experiments, the intervention can be simply stated. If we are testing batteries, for example, we can compare alkaline with carbon, and so the "treatment" is well specified. Or we may want to reduce the variance[1] in our experiment by defining the treatments in terms of alkaline batteries made by specific companies compared with similarly specified carbon batteries. Even in this simple example, however, the choice of how the intervention is defined is important. If the decision maker has only the option of selecting alkaline or carbon batteries, then it may be best to just evaluate the two options: alkaline versus carbon. If, in this situation, we choose "treatment" by brand name, the results of the evaluation may be useless to the decision maker unless we are also able to tell the probabilities of receiving each brand of battery given the choice.

Mental health services are obviously much more complex than batteries. Most interventions have many different facets that must be addressed before an intervention is fully specified. These include the following:

- **Covered Services.** Most managed mental health benefit programs have specific limits on covered services. Managed mental health companies work with a number of different clients with different covered benefits. Some plans may not cover prescription drugs, and others may not offer a continuum of benefits, such as partial hospitalization or intensive outpatient services.

- **Coverage Limits.** Many benefit plans have specific limits on the amount of services that can be provided (30 days of inpatient care), the frequency of services (not more than 2 psychotherapy visits per week), or total benefit costs (not more than $5,000 per year).

- **Reimbursement Strategies.** The proliferation of provider networks and contracting has greatly complicated the task of paying for care. There is a wide variety of payment methods and rates as well as options of whether to use in or out-of-network providers.

- **Authorized Providers.** Different benefit programs have different rules for which providers will be approved for payment. Some will pay marriage and family counselors while others will not. Some will pay only if the care is supervised by a physician.

- **Managed Care Services.** There are a wide variety of managed care services that may be offered, i.e., preadmission review, continued stay review, outpatient review, case management, provider profiling,

---

1. See the "Using Models and Theory" section below for approaches to reduce variance.

on-site audits and records review. Most managed care programs offer some or all of these, depending upon which the client[2] wishes to purchase.

- **Screening Criteria.** The screening criteria are an important facet of most managed care programs. The content of the screens and the way they are applied can vary substantially across programs.
- **Administrative Processes.** Administrative processes are very important to the success of managed mental health programs. They may include claims processing, training of utilization review staff, information systems, reporting, and appeals processing.

These are only some of the factors that may be included in defining the managed care intervention. It may be possible to simply define the intervention as "Company Plan A," where the Plan is one of the packages of services that the managed care company sells. Even with this approach, it is useful to clearly and completely document the various facets of the intervention for future reference. If an evaluation covers a long period of time, it is probable that some aspects of it will change during the evaluation, and it may be critical to know what the changes are.

Each managed mental health program includes some or all of the components discussed above (Brown, Smith and Coulam, 1990). The most basic evaluation question has to do with the effect of managed versus no managed care. The particular managed care program to be evaluated is most likely restricted to the one offered by the firm being evaluated. It might be briefly defined as follows:

- **Covered Services:** The plan covers all acute inpatient care, residential treatment center care for children, partial hospitalization, and outpatient services. The plan also pays for prescription drugs. Other services may be authorized upon the recommendation of a case manager.
- **Coverage Limits:** There are no coverage limits for care preauthorized by the managed mental health program. For care not preauthorized, the limit is 15 days of acute inpatient care and 20 outpatient visits. Residential care and partial hospitalization are not covered without preauthorization. Substance abuse treatment is limited to one 30-day episode per year with a three episode lifetime limit. Outpatient visits are limited to two per week.

---

2. The client here is the employer or third party payor who is purchasing managed mental health services.

- **Reimbursement:** All care is reimbursed on a fee-for-service basis. The provider collects a copayment of $10 per outpatient visit and $35 per inpatient day from the patient. The plan reimburses both network and non-network providers according to a published fee schedule. In addition, network providers participate in a profit sharing plan of up to 15% of the fee schedule amount.
- **Authorized Providers:** Licensed psychiatrists, psychologists and clinical social workers can be reimbursed as independent providers of outpatient, residential, and partial hospitalization services. A psychiatrist must supervise acute inpatient services. There is a provider network, but patients are not required to use it.
- **Managed Care Services:** The managed mental health program requires preauthorization for all acute inpatient, residential, and partial hospitalization admissions. Outpatient treatment is subject to review after the 12th visit. The program also provides continued stay review and discharge planning. Case management is available for exceptional cases upon recommendation of a case reviewer. All review is done by licensed professionals. The utilization review process includes three levels of review with the third level performed by a psychiatrist. All review is done by telephone. The reviewers generally collect information for the review from the attending practitioner. Once a case is referred for case management, the case manager interacts directly with the patient.
- **Screening Criteria:** The utilization review criteria used are the "Company Criteria." In this description, the points at which criteria were revised would have to be specified.
- **Administrative Services:** The program provides basic inquiry services for both plan enrollees and providers. Enrollees are encouraged to use network providers and are referred directly to such providers, if possible. The program provides authorization information to the claims processor but does not process claims directly.

This set of definitions gives a sense of a few of the important parameters that should be specified. It would be reasonable to expect different results from a managed care program that requires patients to use network providers from the one above that allows freedom of choice. If a managed mental health company provides services to several different employer groups and some have freedom of choice while others do not, it is important to account for this difference in the analysis. Similarly, different results are likely if, for example, a plan has limited benefits, does not cover partial hospitalization, or has control over claims processing.

As managed mental health programs mature, it will become increasingly important to evaluate more narrow program alternatives. It may become important, for example, to isolate the effects of the provider network or to use alternative screening criteria and evaluate their effects on cost or utilization. In such cases, it is best if all aspects of the program remain the same except for the particular change being measured. The important point here is that the results of the evaluation, the differences between the control group and the treatment group, are attributable to the intervention. If the intervention includes multiple factors, it will not be possible to isolate the effects of a change on a single factor.

Another important consideration in defining the managed mental health intervention is its timing. For some programs, this is easy because there is a clearly defined start date, the system is fully operational on that date, and the system stays relatively stable over the entire data collection period. For most programs, however, there is often a transitional phase during which new staff are hired, beneficiaries and providers are told about the new program, and current systems are expanded to accept the new workload. Periods of transition can greatly influence the opportunity for an evaluator to collect data on intervention effects. Developing a careful time line to describe the benefit changes and sentinel dates relative to implementation is very helpful.

Stating the Evaluation Questions

The correct evaluation questions must be framed before it is possible to determine the appropriate evaluation design, the best models for analyzing results, and the appropriate data to collect. Caution must be taken with regard to the formulation of evaluation questions. The answers to one set of questions generally lead to new questions that require answers. In almost all cases, new questions will arise that are important, but cannot be answered with the data that were collected for the current evaluation. As the evaluation questions are developed, there is a trade-off between the expense and time required to collect and analyze additional data and not being able to answer all the important questions. The best evaluations are generally those that are designed to answer a few, well formulated, important questions.

Some of the basic evaluation questions in managed mental health include: "Did the introduction of the managed care program (the intervention) reduce the total cost (outcome measure) of mental health benefits?" If the answer to this question is "Yes," the next question may be, "Did the intervention affect certain categories of patients (e.g., children) or certain types of care (e.g., acute inpatient) more than others?" For all questions, the intervention is the same. The questions isolate different categories of effects and characteristics of the system that relate to those effects.

In some cases, the questions may be designed to compare two or more different interventions. "Was the managed care program that restricted patients to network providers more effective than the one that allowed freedom of provider choice?

This chapter generally discusses evaluation in terms of a managed mental health intervention versus no intervention. The approach here is essentially the same for an evaluation that compares two different types of interventions. The basic difference is that the comparisons are made between intervention A and intervention B rather than between the intervention and the control.

Most evaluation questions fall into six general categories. These are cost and utilization questions, quality of care, patient/enrollee satisfaction, outcome, feasibility and provider questions.

Cost and Utilization Questions

These questions are usually concerned with whether the intervention reduced the cost, quantity, or mix of services provided to the enrolled population. In formulating such questions, perspective is important. Did the intervention, for example, reduce the employer's total cost or just the payment for benefits? From the perspective of the managed mental health firm, this important question may concern the administrative costs associated with alternative utilization review programs and the relative effectiveness of these programs in controlling utilization and costs.

When managed mental health programs are first implemented, it may be relatively easy to achieve significant savings when compared to no managed care. As the managed care programs mature, however, and the "fat" is pushed out of the system, it may become more and more difficult to justify the administrative costs of the managed care program. At present, the questions focus on benefit costs and utilization; in the future, the questions may shift to administrative efficiency.

In examining cost and utilization questions, it is useful to factor the total cost equation into meaningful components. The basic equation is:

$$\text{COST}_{\text{Total}} = \text{ELIGIBLES} \times \frac{\text{USERS}}{\text{ELIGIBLE}} \times \frac{\text{UNITS}_{\text{Service}}}{\text{USERS}} \times \frac{\text{COST}}{\text{UNIT}_{\text{Service}}}$$

The first factor in this equation is the number of eligible persons, enrollees, covered lives, or other designation for the number of people who are covered by the program. The number of eligibles is the totality of persons who can be affected by the managed care program. Generally, it is best to count the individuals who are eligible. Some programs do not have good ongoing data on the number of individuals and either settle for the number of families or assume the number of enrollees is constant.

The next factor in this equation, the number of users compared to those who are eligible, is important to determine whether the managed care program is restricting access and whether the utilization rates are normal for the eligible population. The units of service per user factor gives a sense of the effects of managed care on utilization. This factor shows the number of units of service provided once someone enters care. For most managed mental health programs, the expectation would be that the units of service per user will be reduced. Another important factor addresses the cost per unit of service. This one helps understand the issues related to negotiated rates and inflation.

In most practical situations, the equation actually used is more complex than the one above. The rate of service use may be categorized by age, gender, benefit plans or other characteristics of the eligible population. The units of service and cost components for inpatient and outpatient services should be separated. All inpatient care may be considered together, or segregated into residential care, detoxification, day programs, and others. It is useful to examine cost factors separately as well as the total cost.

Quality of Care Questions

As with any significant change in the provision of mental health services, quality of care is of major interest. Without fail, those who oppose managed care point to quality as one of their major criticisms. This criticism is often illustrated by anecdotes about risks to quality due to failure of the managed mental health firm to authorize additional hospitalization. Concerns are expressed about the "moral" dilemma of a practitioner who believes such care is needed, but the utilization reviewer will not agree to pay for it.

These and other quality of care questions are difficult to evaluate. In general, evaluations deal with the effects of interventions on averages— average utilization rates, average cost per patient, average quality of care. But concern about the effects of managed mental health (and managed care in general) on quality is not so much about averages as about specific cases. Even if the evaluation demonstrates that average quality improves under managed mental health, the problem of the depressed teenager whose condition gets worse after additional hospitalization is denied is not resolved to the critics' satisfaction.

Employers, third party payors and managed mental health firms are not yet committed to make available the considerable resources necessary to implement good evaluation studies of the quality of care. Nor is the state of the art sufficiently developed that such studies could be done with a high level of confidence in their outcomes. In evaluating managed mental health programs, the greatest criticism is that care is not authorized at a high enough level for the patient's condition. To evaluate quality, one relatively simple approach would be to look at an available measure of patient functioning or at clinical assessments such as need for close observation or suicidal ideation, and compare these with the treatment setting in which these patients are placed.

Two particularly difficult problems in trying to evaluate quality are:

- It is difficult to find data on the quality of care provided prior to the implementation of the managed care program, so there is no baseline.
- The quality and availability of information on outpatients create a problem. In order to find patients who have been denied access to inpatient services that they perhaps should have received, one must look at patients in the outpatient setting. It is often very difficult to obtain access to outpatient records, and even when they are available, the quality of the information is generally poor.

It is important, but difficult, to evaluate the quality of service under managed mental health programs. While it may be possible to formulate and answer questions about average quality of care, such answers are not likely to satisfy critics who use individual case examples to argue against managed mental health programs.

Patient/Enrollee Questions

Patient satisfaction and the effects of various interventions on patient access to care and on adverse selection of health benefit programs are important questions to address. Most evaluations of them rely on patient satisfaction surveys, or analysis of inquiry volumes and content for answers.

Client Outcome Questions

One very difficult area to deal with in the evaluation of managed mental health programs has to do with outcomes—the effect of the intervention on the patient's ability to function, quality of life, or general well-being. The difficulty lies in the problems of measuring outcomes and also with defining the intervention adequately enough to allow the changes to be adequately attributed to the intervention. There is growing pressure for more outcome oriented studies in mental health that rigorously evaluate the effectiveness of different treatment protocols. These studies can be very helpful in defining managed care screening criteria and establishing norms of care. In general, it is difficult to justify the costs of comprehensive outcome evaluations to assess the effects of managed mental health programs.

Feasibility Questions

Many important evaluation questions revolve around the administrative feasibility of implementing and running a managed mental health program. Some of the questions may be related to the reactions of the professional community to proposed changes in documentation requirements. In the Department of Defense Norfolk Demonstration Project (CHAMPUS), for example, there was tremendous resistance to the requirement to submit outpatient records for quality review. Other examples include issues related to qualifications of staff to perform certain functions, time required to collect information for utilization review, and ability to develop provider networks in certain areas or with certain contract provisions.

Provider Questions

The effects of managed mental health on providers are very important to most evaluations, and these effects can be very complex. Issues include administrative burden, changes in practice patterns, market shares, provider incomes and profitability. These questions can be difficult to deal with in evaluation studies because, in the long term, provider behavior is likely to change in order to adapt to whatever system is put into place. If the managed care program does a good job of reducing the level of care for adolescents, for example, it is likely that some inpatient programs will shut down. In such an environment there may be less competition, and as a result, the price per unit of service may go up. Thus, while the short-term effects may be good, in the long-term they may be less so.

Once an evaluation question is formulated, the next step is to determine what it really means and how its effects can be measured. It is often difficult to get past this hurdle, and so questions must be reformulated before it is possible to develop measures. Consider, for example, the question: Did the managed mental health intervention change provider practice patterns? To answer this question, a practice pattern must first be defined in such a way that allows it to be described quantitatively. To illustrate, consider a practice pattern for an episode of care that is defined as the "four-tuple" (number of inpatient days, number of residential treatment center days, number of partial hospitalization days, number of outpatient visits). Questions arise as to whether the number of admissions, use of drugs, frequency of visits, and order in which the services are provided should be included. Even with the relatively simple four-tuple, it is difficult to define a change and even more difficult to decide what constitutes a good versus a bad change. Using just the four-tuple, it would be appropriate to expect that care would move from inpatient and residential toward partial hospitalization and outpatient due to the implementation of managed care. Then independent variables such as diagnosis, patient age and sex, location, and intervention/nonintervention would be used to determine which are important for discriminating among different practice patterns.

Basic Outcome Evaluation Problems

The purpose of an outcome evaluation is to measure the effects of the intervention. Outcomes may include days of inpatient care as well as admission and recidivism rates. While it is relatively easy to measure trends, it is difficult to do so for effects that can be safely attributed to the intervention, to compare what happened with what would have happened in the absence of that intervention. The critical problem is, of course, with estimating what "would have happened" without the intervention. There are several ways of making such estimates. This is the central problem of evaluation design.

To illustrate the problem and several design options, assume that we are trying to evaluate the effects of a managed mental health program on inpatient hospital days per user. Here the measurement problem is fairly straight forward—we will simply take the ratio of the number of hospital days and the number of users of mental health services for any given period of time. The problem of being able to attribute an observed change to the intervention is best solved by taking the pool of eligible persons and randomizing them into two groups: one getting access to the new benefit (treatment) and the other remaining with the conventional benefit plan (control). The control becomes the vehicle for measuring what would have happened without the intervention. After some follow up period, the difference in inpatient days per user between the groups would be the estimate of the program outcome.

Things other than the managed care intervention may influence the number of inpatient days per user for the control group. These confounding influences affect the degree of certainty with which the measured effect can be attributed to the intervention. Such influences may include the providers used, severity of illness, age, gender, and living arrangements. With a randomized design, however, it is assumed that these are randomly distributed across both groups. Hence, with this design, any significant difference in observed use rates can be attributed to the intervention since the intervention is the only factor that systematically differs between the groups.

Randomized studies are not easy to conduct. Often there are significant political or ethical problems with withholding certain services from one group. Also, it can be administratively very difficult to allocate services differently to individual patients who are randomly assigned to different treatments. In such cases, it may be feasible to randomize families, different employee groups or different demographic areas. Once we get away from simple randomization, the designs, the analysis, and the risks become much more complex. While detailed discussion of the many different approaches to randomized designs is beyond the scope of this chapter, there are many excellent approaches to randomization that can be considered.

Aside from randomization, there are other ways to estimate program effects and other threats to safely attributing those effects to the intervention.[3]

The evaluator must rely on more explicit effects to quantify and adjust for potentially confounding factors and must be sensitive to the types of threats imposed by alternate designs in drawing conclusions. If, for instance, a before-after design is used, the program effect is measured as the difference between the period before the managed care program was implemented and the period following its implementation. The concern here about attribution is whether other factors such as practice patterns, seasonal effects, and aging of the patients changed from one period to the next and caused some or all of the measured changes in inpatient days per user. Since changes in technology, reimbursement, and supply factors are so persistent in health care, such research designs are considered weak. Hence, proper attribution of measured effects to any particular intervention is difficult. If such designs must be used because of data availability constraints, the best protection is a long baseline period, coupled with as long a follow-up period as possible. The long baseline[4] allows a better estimate of what would have happened absent the intervention than would a shorter one.

Graphically, this can be illustrated easily (see Figure 1). With a simple pre-post test, data are collected at time 4 before the intervention (point A), and time 7 after the intervention (point B). The difference in admission rates is A minus B, which we could use as a program effect if we are willing to assume that point A is an approximation of "what would have happened at point B if there had been no intervention." Alternatively, if we add data for times 1, 2, and 3, (a longer baseline period) we can construct a better estimate of "what would have happened at point B if we had not intervened." Using regression techniques, we can estimate the line xx (Draper and Smith, 1966). We then predict that our study population would have had inpatient use rates equal to A1 at time 7, and we would use A1 minus B as our program effect estimate. In the example, we say that the difference between A and B has two parts. One part is the continuing downward trend in admission rates (A to A1), and the other part is our program effect.

Of course, there are other things that could have changed between

---

3. For an excellent review of design options and threats to validity, see Campbell, Donald T., and Stanley, Julian C., "Experimental and Quasi-Experimental Designs for Research on Teaching," in Gage, N.L. (Ed.), *Handbook of Research on Teaching* (Chicago, Rand McNally & Co., 1963).

4. Using regression models with trend factors.

times 4 and 7 that would confound our interpretation of A1 minus B as the result of the managed care intervention. Estimating such things and noting the kinds of influences they might have had on the outcome is helpful. In the end, however, before/after designs are weak and there is the risk of incorrectly attributing change (or the lack of it) to the intervention.

Similarly, there are designs that compare two different populations: one group affected by the intervention, and one that is not. These could be two cities or counties, two different payor populations, etc. Direct comparison of the treated and reference populations presumes that the latter emulates "what would have happened" to the study group had it not been treated. Significant variations in health care practice patterns across areas and variations in practice styles across providers make such designs difficult to defend. Basically, the implied program effect is confounded by any and all things that may be different between groups.

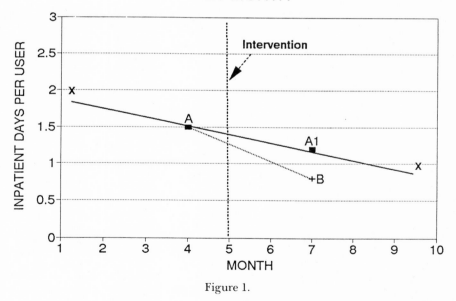

Figure 1.

A more promising evaluation approach for managed mental health combines the pre-post and study-comparison approaches. Here, the trend in the reference group is used to approximate what the trend would be in

the study group. The balance of the pre-post change in the study becomes
the estimated program effect. Graphically (Figure 2) the change in the
inpatient days for the study group (A→Bs) is partitioned into the trend
part and the treatment effect part. The trend is observed in the reference
population. The value Bs (estimated from the trend As→Bs which is
parallel to the trend As→Bs) then becomes our estimate of what would
have happened in the study group had there not been an intervention.
The difference between Bs and Bs is the estimated program effect. This
estimate may be wrong, but it is subject to fewer threats of validity than
either the pre-post or study-comparison group designs alone. For a
factor to confound the result, it would have to be present in one group
and not in the other *and* would have had to change at the same time as
the intervention.

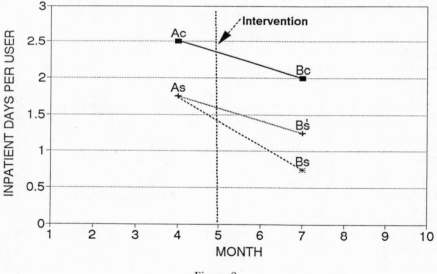

INPATIENT DAYS PER USER
BY MONTH

Figure 2.

In our evaluation of the Department of Defense managed mental
health demonstration in Norfolk, Virginia, we used a variation of this
pre-post, study-comparison group design. We collected claims data for
Norfolk, San Diego, and the United States for the 24-month period
before and 30 months during the demonstration. The last eight months

of claims data for San Diego were not available because of changes in the program for California beginning in August 1988 (Smith and Coulam, 1988). Figures 3 and 4 show the number of inpatient days per user by month and the cost per inpatient day by month.[5] The managed care program became effective in October 1986. Figure 4 shows an obvious, large reduction in the cost per inpatient day as a result of the demonstration project. The effect on number of days per user is much less clear. The Norfolk data show a downward trend which brings it below both the San Diego and the national rates. This trend, however, began before the managed care program and the only significant change that began after the demonstration is the change in slope beginning in August 1988. We had hypothesized a change at this point because the managed care firm initiated a new utilization review committee beginning in August 1988; thus we feel comfortable attributing the change in slope to the committee. When we began this analysis, we planned to use annual data, but the annual data did not allow us to isolate the hypothesized effects of the mid-year change. This illustrates two important points. First, it is important to clearly document the intervention. We had to know that the utilization review process changed in August 1988 in order to hypothesize that utilization rates might change as a result. Second, the period of aggregation for the data can make a difference in the ability of the evaluation to find program effects.

Another important point about data can be derived from Figure 3. Note that the data for both the national and Norfolk series appear to have a downward trend at the end of the data collection period. This downward trend can be practically attributed to the fact that we were relying on claims data for the analysis, and we only collected data on claims submitted through June 1989. We know that there were about $300,000 in claims paid by the Norfolk contractor during the period, July–September; however, we suspect that the national data are less complete than the Norfolk data because there was a lot of pressure on providers in Norfolk to submit their claims quickly. This means that we cannot attribute all of the decrease at the end of the period to the demonstration.

The design type that is chosen does not guarantee success. All outcome evaluations are hypothesis testing activities to try to demonstrate the existence of change. As such, the concern is not only about having a

---

5. Figures 3, 4, 5, 8, 9 and 10 originate from Coulam and Smith (1990).

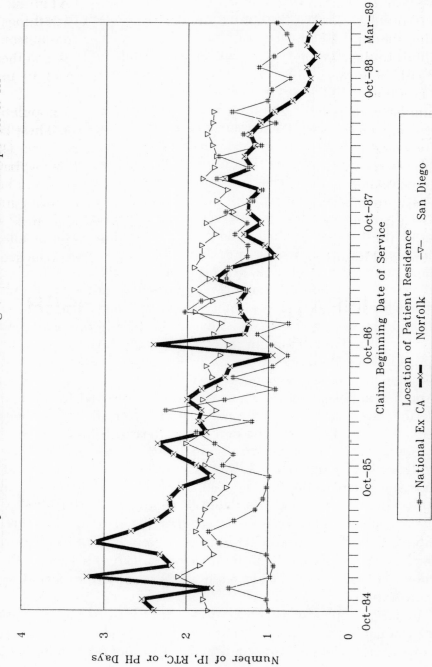

Figure 3.

NUMBER OF DAYS (IP, RTC, PH) PER USER BY MONTH
Comparison of Norfolk, San Diego, and National Except CA & HI

Location of Patient Residence

—#— National Ex CA   —×— Norfolk   —▽— San Diego

Source: CHAMPUS Claims Data Processed Through June 1989
         National Data Excludes Claims from California and Hawaii

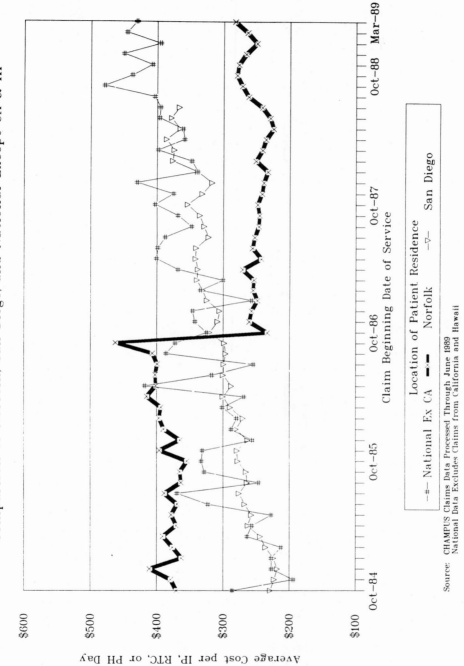

Figure 4.

COST PER DAY (IP, RTC, PH)
Comparison of Norfolk, San Diego, and National Except CA & HI

Source: CHAMPUS Claims Data Processed Through June 1989
National Data Excludes Claims from California and Hawaii

valid explanation of what happened to the study group, but also about whether the observed change could have been due to chance alone. There are many factors such as patient health status, exposure to stress, and provider/patient interaction that are outside the control of the evaluator but can affect the number of inpatient days for a patient. Such independent factors cause variations in the outcome measure (inpatient days per user) that are unrelated to the treatment. In light of these factors (the "noise"), the important question is: "Is the measured program effect large enough to be isolated from the normal variations caused by these external factors?" Obviously, the answer depends on how much "noise" exists, how large the program effect is, and how much statistical power[6] is provided by the experimental design being used. The statistical power can be improved by increasing the sample size. The issue here is that with any design, even a randomized trial, there is a controllable chance that small true effects of a program will be rejected as insignificant. For a particular design, the probability that this will happen increases as the "noise" increases or the size of the intervention effect decreases.

As a part of any evaluation design, the evaluator must do a detailed power analysis to determine whether or not the design will allow expected program effects to be discovered. If the power is not adequate, there are two general strategies to increase power. First, increasing the sample size increases the power so one should strive for the largest possible sample. There are trade-offs, however, between sample size, cost of the evaluation, and the quality and extent of the data collected on each patient. Second, reducing the variance of the "noise" increases the power. There are various methods of using sophisticated designs or modelling techniques to reduce the variance and increase the power without increasing the sample size. In analyzing the effects of managed care on inpatient days per user, for example, it may be possible to build a predictive model of inpatient utilization that explains some portion of the normal variations among patients. The model may consider factors such as age, gender, occupation, or health status. The use of such models, even within randomized studies, can reduce unexplained variation in the outcome

---

6. Statistical power is a measure of the level of assurance that the experimenter will find an intervention effect if it exists. For example, the power of an experiment might be stated: If the intervention reduces the number of inpatient days per user by 10% or more, there is a 90% probability you will conclude that the intervention had an effect. A good reference text on power analysis is Jacob Cohen, *Statistical Power Analysis for the Behavioral Sciences.* New York: Academic Press, 1977.

measure and increase the power of the design to detect small program effects.

Using Models and Theory

A consequence of non-random evaluation designs is the difficulty of properly interpreting findings. In evaluations of managed mental health programs, this problem is further complicated by multiple outcomes that usually are of interest including changes in cost and utilization of mental health services, in use of non-mental health services, in patient outcomes and/or in the quality of care. Even with a strong design, the multiplicity of outcomes can yield a pattern of implied effects that is confusing if they are not internally consistent. In weaker designs, there is a reluctance to rely on a particular outcome as proof that an intervention worked but more comforting if there is a pattern of effects (including qualitative findings) consistent with what would have been anticipated if the interventions were working as expected.

All evaluations, regardless of design, will profit from a carefully thought out description of the patterns of anticipated effects across various outcomes and various patient types. These prior expectations help in three ways. First, just the process of thinking through the possible effects of the intervention helps to understand the dynamics of the situation and insures that the correct factors are being looked at. Second, the anticipated effects form the basis for stating hypotheses about which and how outcomes should change. Third, the theory becomes the yardstick that can be used to interpret the results. If the collection of actual changes matches the expected changes, then there is comfort with the findings. If, on the other hand, there are differences between expected and actual outcomes, the theory did not hold up and the possible effects that could be caused by the intervention must be reformulated.

If we were evaluating the effects of adding partial hospitalization as a covered service under a managed mental health program, for example, we might hypothesize the following effects:

Measure	Expectation about the effect of a partial hospitalization benefit
Hospital Admission Rates	Decrease
Inpatient Days for Persons with xxxx.x Diagnosis	No Change
Inpatient Days for Persons with yyyy.y Diagnosis	Decrease
Residential Treatment Center Days for Adolescents with	

zzzz.z Diagnosis	Decrease
Outpatient Visits	No Change
Total Costs of Care	Decrease

We could also make more detailed specifications such as: we expect that partial hospitalization days will be substituted for acute inpatient days or residential days at a rate of about 1.5 partial per inpatient day. Once we have stated our expectations, we can examine the data and determine whether or not the results match the expectations. If we notice, for instance, that apparent program effects on inpatient days for *both* xxxx.x and yyyy.y are down, we may worry that some factor other than our intervention was confounding the evaluation; or that our utilization review screens for partial hospitalization are not adequately discriminating among different types of cases.

Theories can be more elaborate than a simple set of prognostications as in the table above. Indeed, social scientists and professional evaluation experts can spend enormous amounts of time trying to work through the logical consequences of particular interventions. This encourages many to avoid theory altogether and get on with the analysis of the data. Better guidance would be to set down some type of theory or expectations about how the program should work to affect outcomes. This can be as simple a task as a couple of brainstorming sessions and can incorporate a quick review of the results of other similar evaluations.

Importance of Descriptive and Baseline Data

Most evaluations depend upon sophisticated statistical techniques to standardize data and isolate program effects. While these methods are essential to assure that the results are true program effects, their value for communicating results to decision makers is limited. Simple means, frequency data, and associated trends are easy to prepare and understand. Descriptive data serve an evaluation in several ways.

The *practical significance* of estimated program effects to decision makers will depend, in part, on whether the results are apparent in raw, unadjusted data. If the basic evaluation outcomes are not visible from raw data, then any significant measured program effects are probably quite small and discernable only by means of statistical adjustment procedures. It is difficult to explain why and how such statistical procedures cause an effect to be discernable from otherwise inconsequential trends or differences in raw data. It is also questionable whether or not program changes need to be made when effects are so small as to not be readily observable.

Consequently, it is prudent to carefully understand the behavior of the important outcome measures over time in study and control groups. If the total cost effect is small, for example, it is important to examine the components of cost. Perhaps the number of users in the treatment group increased much faster than the number of users in the control group. This increase may offset the decreased cost per user in the treatment group. The focus can then be on what caused the increase in the number of users and whether this increase is a good outcome (e.g., indicating improved access to care) or a bad outcome (e.g., the result of providers generating unnecessary utilization to preserve income). The ability to respond to this question may be very important to the decision to implement a program or redesign it.

This example is particularly relevant to the evaluation of some managed mental health programs. When we analyzed the data for the Norfolk demonstration, we noticed a substantial increase in the number of people using mental health services. We hypothesized that the publicity about the program's implementation had made the beneficiaries more aware of their benefit and how to access it. This increased awareness would lead to a higher number of users. Once the data for Norfolk, San Diego, and the national sample were available, we plotted the number of users per 1000 eligible persons each month. The plot is shown in Figure 5 below. Surprisingly, the trend proved not significantly different in Norfolk. This result tells us that the use rate is increasing throughout the nation, and it tells us that the implementation of the managed mental health program did not significantly affect the increase.

Another important point that can be made from these data is the importance of control or comparison groups. These groups help to provide baseline data that can be important to explain the outcomes. Without such data, it is very difficult to assess the effects of the intervention.

In the implementation of most managed mental health programs, it is often difficult to get an acceptable baseline. Usually, when employers implement such a program, they do so for all employees. For this example, if we eliminate everything except the Norfolk data—a situation similar to implementing a managed care program for all employees—the answer changes. The change in the user rate increases with the demonstration. Without the baseline data, we would have been led to believe that the managed care program intervention increased the number

Figure 5.

NUMBER OF MENTAL HEALTH USERS PER 1000 ELIGIBLE PERSONS BY MONTH
Comparison of Norfolk, San Diego, and National Except CA & HI

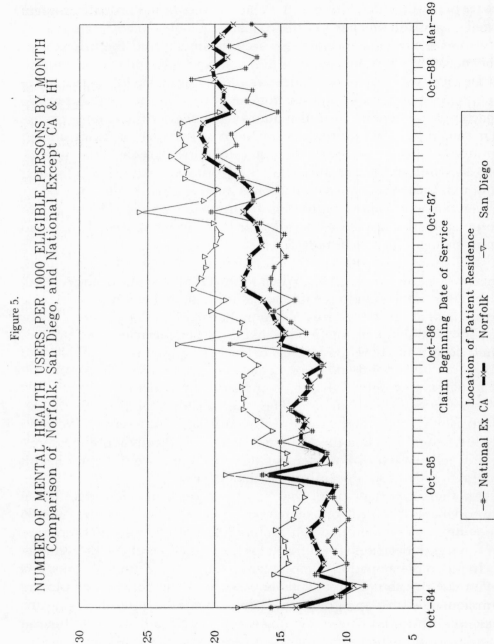

Source: CHAMPUS Claims Data Processed Through June 1989
          National Data Excludes Claims from California and Hawaii

of users per eligible. This still does not tell us whether such an increase would be considered good or bad. This answer depends upon the objectives of the program and cannot be answered based solely upon the use rate data.[7]

Descriptive analysis of *distribution data* is particularly important in understanding certain types of interventions because the intervention may impact differentially on patients with different characteristics—e.g., age, gender, severity of illness. The effects of the intervention on means or averages, while crucial, often obfuscate crucial textural effects. These subsidiary nuances are often the source of information on *how* the program works and on what may be done to improve it.

For example, Figures 6 and 7 illustrate a home care case management intervention in upstate and downstate New York sites. The statistical results found that the program saved dollars upstate but resulted in higher spending downstate. Figure 6 shows a frequency distribution on total health care spending per client month in upstate sites, and Figure 7 shows the same data for the downstate areas. Each figure plots the frequencies by cost category for the intervention groups and the control groups. These raw data tell the story about why the same program had much different consequences in the two regions. The simple figures show:

- That downstate (Figure 7), the intervention moved a large fraction of very low cost cases into mid-range spending categories; that is, the program provided home care services to a large number of persons who otherwise would not have consumed many health care resources.
- That upstate (Figure 6), this effect was more modest.
- That downstate, the intervention had little apparent effect on the frequency of high cost cases (right tail of the distribution).
- That upstate, there was a discernable shift toward reducing the frequency of cases costing $1,600–$3,000 per month.

We could speculate, from these simple frequencies, that the upstate program was more cost effective because of more successful *substitution* of modest cost home care for higher cost nursing home care. Downstate,

---

7. If one's objective is to reduce total cost, then increase in users would be considered bad unless we could show that use of mental health services reduced use of non-mental health services, reduced absenteeism, etc. On the other hand, if the objective is to provide a better health benefit, the increase may be considered positive, provided it can be shown that the new users needed services.

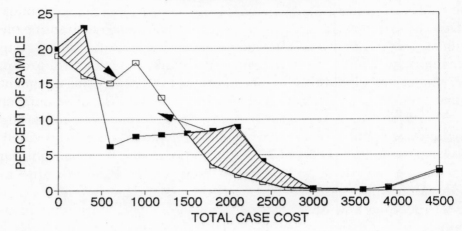

Figure 6.

there is evidence that augmentation of services dominates substitution. This type of analysis is particularly relevant to managed care type programs that are expected to affect the high cost cases more than the low cost ones.

This type of analysis is not a substitute for more rigorous hypotheses testing using standardization. But it may, in the end, be quite helpful in explaining the results to audiences not readily conversant with statistics.

Choosing Sensitive Measures

The imperfection of evaluation research designs and measures creates significant problems of unexplained variability in health and mental health evaluation outcome measures. The statistical "noise" often masks small but important effects of programs. The noise is a product of:

- Significant person to person differences in health and health care seeking behaviors that cannot be measured and controlled in evaluation work.
- Significant "bluntness" in measures of outcome; for example, to

DISTRIBUTION OF COST PER CASE
Downstate New York Sites

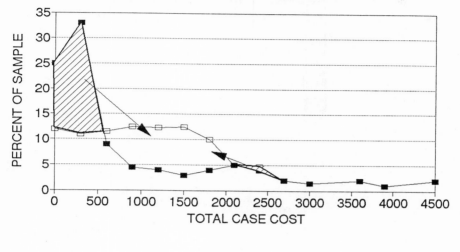

Figure 7.

measure improvements in function or quality of life, extreme and insensitive outcomes like death or readmission rates must often be used.

- Significant presence of interactions between the intervention and client characteristics; these interactions imply differing program effects on subgroups of clients (groups like the old, those who live alone, with high prior use, with specific diagnoses, etc.). Thus, measured program effects often become an average of an amalgam of different effects, possibly of opposite direction.

Careful attention to choosing measures and samples can improve the evaluator's ability to obtain better resolution on program effects. This is most critical when primary data collection is prohibitively expensive and secondary data must be used. Several techniques can be used to improve "signal-to-noise" ratios in mental health evaluation work. These include:

Tracer Cases. Very often, sampling strategies focus attention on only one or more very specific type of case. This may be a particular diagnosis, a particular problem, or some functional limitation. The reason for such a narrow focus is that measurement of the critical *determinants* of outcome (cost, use, or quality) are too poor to be able to pool case types together without generating large unexplained outcome variations. Choosing a narrow band of cases is one way of controlling the unmeasurable differences in outcomes across case types.

Use of selected tracers will limit "noise" and probably improve the precision of effect estimates. In general, their use may eliminate risks of spurious results and improve the validity of the work. Use of tracers, however, does not allow generalization to all cases. That is, it cannot know what the overall effects of the program are nor can it be certain that choosing other "tracers" would have resulted in similar results. Hence, tracer work is usually a complement to, not a substitute for, a general sampling strategy. The tracer results may help to corroborate general work where there would be worry about the consequences of poor measurement of prognostic factors.

In managed mental health, individuals with a specific range in level of functioning could be looked at with a measure such as the GAS score. This would be true as well for a specific diagnosis or type of condition on which managed care could be expected to have a significant effect—for example, adolescents with a depression diagnosis.

In the CHAMPUS project, episodes of care for adolescents with a depression diagnosis were analyzed (Smith and Coulam, 1989). The results showed that adolescents with depression were, on average, almost five times as costly as any other group, and that the managed care intervention was very effective in reducing the cost for this group. We were concerned, however, with the validity of the analysis because we found that patients who had been receiving care for a long period of time tended to have multiple diagnoses; a depression diagnosis may be a consequence of long term mental health care rather than a useful criterion for patient classification.

Care Sensitive Tracers. Sometimes tracers can be selected because of the belief that the effects will be largest or easiest to see given the blunt outcome measures that are available. If such "probable high impact tracers" can be identified, there is a better chance to improve the "signal-to-noise" problem. If we *fail* to see the predicted outcome in these cases, we may be able to reason that effects do not exist in the aggregate. If we *do* find a significant program effect for such cases, we cannot know how pervasive the result is among the others.

How are these cases selected? Assume that we are trying to detect changes in quality of care after the introduction of a major managed mental health program that has significantly reduced the number of authorizations for inpatient care. However, we only have patient mortality[8] as a potential quality marker and mortality is obviously a very blunt (though potentially important) measure, i.e., "quality" can fall alarmingly for many types of patients without much change in the mortality rate. In addition, much of the outcome variation is likely due to severity (which we cannot measure well) and practitioner competence (which is not likely to be directly related to budget). In trying to select a tracer to evaluate mortality, the following questions would arise:

- Can we select a set of case types where the blunt outcome (in this case death) is not a rare event?
- Can we select a set of case types where the intervention is likely to be best related to the blunt outcome?

Which resources do administrators have control of that, if changed, may have a material life risk for patients? Which types of cases would these resources tend to compromise? Expert panels could be used to answer such questions, yielding a set of tracers. As constructed, they would be cases carefully tailored to the specific intervention and to the available measures.

Choosing Denominators. In analyzing utilization and cost measures of outcomes, it is often difficult to confidently interpret the pattern array of concepts such as costs per day, days per stay, and admission rates. Part of the problem arises because those getting care are subject to trends (or local practice variations) in technology and severity. So when admission rates, costs per day, lengths of stay, and costs of stay are examined between study and comparison groups, we worry about comparing apples to apples. With case management interventions, of particular concern are measures of cost or use of particular services, since we are often

---

8. Perhaps we should just examine the suicide rate; however, the classification of a death as suicide is not generally reliable. And the deaths may not get reported to the program unless special efforts are made to collect this information.

deliberately trying to intervene in the selection processes that determine "who gets particular types of care."

One useful vehicle to consider is to state outcome measures in per capita, per eligible or per eligible person month terms whenever possible. This differs from measures using denominators such as per user, per stay, or per episode of care. The per capita/eligible person measures internalize any and all treatment effects on the fraction of persons getting care and any resultant effects on the severity of users. Hence, such measures of cost or use provide bottom-line program effects.

In analyzing the Norfolk data and comparing it with the San Diego and national data, we first divided by the number of eligible persons to get number of users per eligible person by month. We defined a user as any individual who had used any type of mental health services during the month. We then examined the average mix of services per user (acute inpatient days per user, residential days per user, outpatient visits per user, etc.). In each case, the user is a user of any services during the period. Within this framework, we were able to examine the relative mix of services provided each user as shown in Figure 8, and we could examine the changes in the user rates for a particular service as shown in Figure 9 for inpatient services.

As indicated by the figures, the change in service mix was quite significant for the Norfolk project. However, if one just looks at the change in services provided to users of that particular service (rather than a mental health user as defined above), the monthly data are relatively stable. This is due in part to the fact that we were looking at monthly rather than longer time periods. For treatment periods that exceed a number of months, the quantity of service provided each month is more a measure of the intensity rather than duration of care.

Consider, for example, residential treatment center care in which the patient may have a length of stay of 180 days or more. The number of days per month for these patients is limited to 30, so we would expect the units of service per user to be near 30 days. If our program were to cut the average length of stay by 30 days, we might not see a big reduction in the intensity. Rather, we would see fewer months of service or a reduction in the number of users by month. This change for residential care is illustrated in Figure 10 below.

Figure 8.

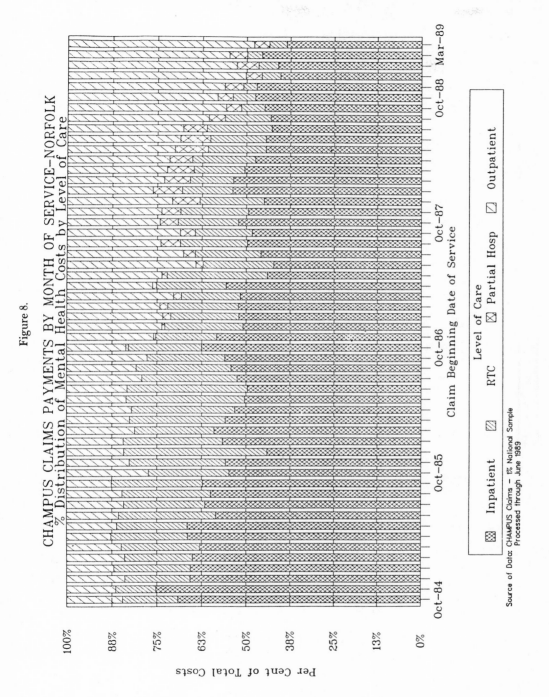

CHAMPUS CLAIMS PAYMENTS BY MONTH OF SERVICE—NORFOLK
% Distribution of Mental Health Costs by Level of Care

Source of Data: CHAMPUS Claims – 1% National Sample
Processed through June 1989

Managed Mental Health Services

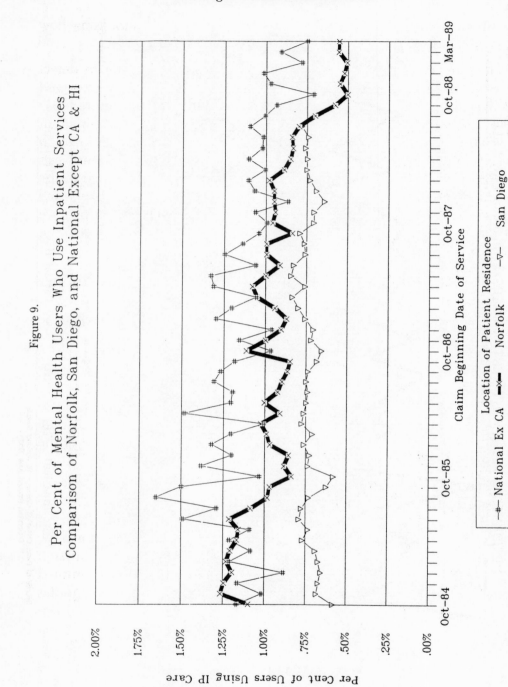

Figure 9.

Per Cent of Mental Health Users Who Use Inpatient Services
Comparison of Norfolk, San Diego, and National Except CA & HI

Source: CHAMPUS Claims Data Processed Through June 1989
National Data Excludes Claims from California and Hawaii

Figure 10.

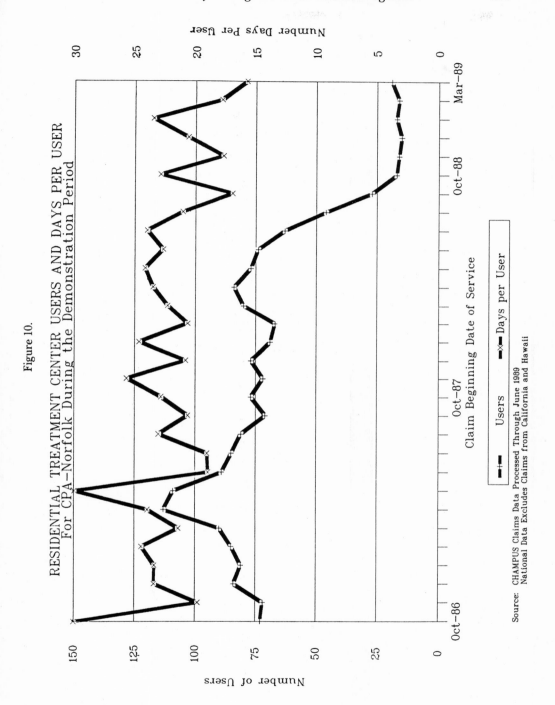

RESIDENTIAL TREATMENT CENTER USERS AND DAYS PER USER
For CPA–Norfolk During the Demonstration Period

Source: CHAMPUS Claims Data Processed Through June 1989
National Data Excludes Claims from California and Hawaii

Summary

This chapter has discussed what the authors consider to be some of the important issues in the evaluation of managed mental health programs as well as the difficulties associated with them. There are many pitfalls in such evaluations and those programs implemented in "real world" environments rather than in a laboratory are particularly difficult to evaluate. It is not possible to do a foolproof evaluation of programs as complex as managed mental health care. Just collecting and analyzing basic data, however, i.e., the number of eligible persons, the number of users by type of service, costs and patient demographics and condition, can lead to very useful information on program performance.

For managed mental health programs, evaluation should be an ongoing process. The programs are constantly evolving over time as is the general health care environment in which they operate. In setting up a basic on-going evaluation strategy, a good starting point is to think about what will be the important questions that clients are likely to ask and that management should have answers to. The next step is to determine what information will be most useful for answering these questions and to design a set of basic reports and analyses that will provide the answers. Some of the ideas discussed in this chapter can be used in this process.

Once it is decided what types of analyses are needed, the issue becomes what data are available to answer the questions. Generally, the data currently available do not suffice and it is necessary to adjust the reports and analyses, and when possible, collect additional data. The availability of data also affects the timing of the analysis. If, for example, claims data are used, it may be months or even years before all of the data are available. If, on the other hand, data available through a concurrent utilization review program are used, it may be possible to analyze very quickly what is expected to happen based upon authorizations. Once the claims data are available, it may be necessary to estimate the differences between authorized care and delivered care, and the differences between estimated costs and actual costs.

Finally, one collects and analyzes data to get a sense of what is changing. While it is critical to use statistically rigorous sampling and analysis techniques, it is also important to understand that we are dealing with operational programs and assessing interventions that influence what is happening in the "real world." Regardless of how rigorous are the evaluation design, sampling, data collection and analysis, it will not be possible to get all the answers and there will be uncertainty associated with those that are obtained.

Evaluations should start off with modest objectives and make use of available data to the extent possible. Careful analysis of available data can help to focus on the important questions, to assess the quality of the data and to develop an improved evaluation design. From such a starting point, it is possible to develop a more comprehensive evaluation program that will be able to meet the needs of the program managers and the clients. Comprehensive evaluations of a program such as managed mental health are very complex and require a great deal of detailed information collected over a long period of time. It is important that the foundation for such programs be well grounded.

REFERENCES

Brown, D.E., Smith, J.C.H. and Coulam, R.: *Applicability of Managed Care Techniques to the Implementation of a DoD Patient Care Management System for Mental Health.* Abt Associates, Cambridge, MA, 1990.

Cambell, D.T. and Stanley, J.C.: Experimental and quasi-experimental designs for research on teaching. In Gage, N.L., ed., *Handbook of Research on Teaching.* Chicago, Rand McNally, 1963.

Cohen, J.: *Statistical Power Analysis for the Behavioral Sciences.* New York, Academic Press, 1977.

Coulam, R. and Smith, J.C.H.: *Evaluation of CPA–Norfolk Demonstration Project: Final Report.* Report submitted pursuant to DoD Contract MDA 906-87-C-0003, Abt Associates, Cambridge, MA, 1990.

Draper, N.R. and Smith, H.: *Applied Regression Analysis.* New York, John Wiley, 1966.

Smith, J.C.H. and Coulam, R.: *Analysis of Deleted Sponsor Groups from the Claims Data Bases for the Evaluation of the CPA–Norfolk Demonstration Project.* Cambridge, MA, Abt Associates, 1988.

Smith, J.C.H. and Coulam, R.: *Evaluation of CPA–Norfolk Demonstration Project: PreDemonstration Mental Health Cost and Utilization in Norfolk and San Diego.* Report submitted pursuant to DoD Contract MDA 906-87-C-0003. Cambridge, MA, Abt Associates, 1989.

Chapter 10

QUALITY ASSURANCE IN
MANAGED MENTAL HEALTH

Jeffrey L. Berlant

Definitions of quality health care cover a wide range. To some, quality is synonymous with "standard care." Legal definitions of professional responsibility for the quality of health care build on the concept of the duty to provide a level of care similar to that of the "average" practitioner. In the past, the standard practice of the average practitioner in the community was used as the benchmark of acceptability for purposes of defining malpractice. Advances in medicine and in communication technology have led to changes in the legal definitions of malpractice, so that national rather than local standards are more commonly used. Expert opinions about innovative or controversial approaches now contribute to definitions of what is accepted as quality as well as the practice of the average practitioner.

Another approach to the definition of quality views it as "not substandard care." Certain practices are defined as "substandard" and are not expected to be used. The application of leeches for fever, or the irradiation of thymus glands in infants would be examples of such practices. Not responding to certain well recognized symptoms or syndromes would also be substandard practice. In this approach, anything outside the realm of recognizable substandard care is considered as quality care. Those practitioners who value very wide latitude in clinical decisions appear to have an affinity for this type of definition.

Another definition views quality as "optimal care," care that is superior to the average. Although not useful as a legal definition of quality, this very common meaning is the stuff of everyday language. Variations on this theme appear in some health care delivery systems that strive to enhance the quality of practice, to design systems of "high quality care," not just "avoid substandard care."

Some quality care definitions build on assumptions about changes that are expected to improve standard practice. Quality as "the application of science," for example, might include ordering extensive laboratory tests to fully delineate a patient's physiological status or the use of highly complex new medical technologies such as transplants, dialysis, or new surgical procedures. Diagnoses and treatments that attempt to apply the findings of biological science are assumed to be superior, even in the absence of evidence of efficacy or cost effectiveness.

The foregoing definitions of quality—"standard practice," "not substandard practice," "optimal care," and "scientific care"—are all based upon a concept of quality as adherence to certain desirable rules of practice. If practitioners follow (or at least do not violate) certain rules or standards, then they are practicing quality medicine, regardless of outcome or other effects.

Other definitions of "quality" look not at whether professional behavior adheres to particular rules of practice but at the *consequences of practice.* One such definition focuses on "consumer (patient and family) satisfaction" as the ultimate arbiter of quality, although few clinicians would substitute this for definitions of quality related to standards of practice. Nonetheless, consumers form their own judgments of what constitutes quality care, and these judgments are important to practitioners, particularly in competitive situations. Adherents of "informed consent" urge greater involvement of patients in medical decision making so that patient goals and values are reflected in treatment plans, thereby broadening the concept of quality.

Quality is also defined as the "avoidance of adverse outcomes," in effect, all practice that does not lead to patient deterioration. Although such an approach appears to be excessively narrow, many hospital quality assurance systems have been constructed around screening for adverse outcomes as a means to eradicate them in the future. The definition focuses on readily defined, undesirable outcomes. Undesirable practices, i.e., those that do not adhere to whatever rules of practice are adopted, are overlooked so long as undesired outcomes do not occur.

Another outcome type definition of quality views quality as "efficacious" care that makes things "better." The use of penicillin for a condition well demonstrated to benefit from it is an example of efficacious care. Within this definition fall two subtypes: efficacious care as defined by "previously demonstrated benefit in similar patients," and efficacious care as defined by "improvement in the patient's condition." Quality care according to this definition encompasses all those practices known to benefit patients;

a high-quality system is one that gets its patients better, irrespective of the means.

Paul Ellwood (1988), an outspoken advocate of quality promotion via the use of systematically gathered information about clinical outcomes, has called for the construction and implementation of a national data base about patients, interventions, and outcomes of treatment. He has proposed that this approach find "the relation between medical interventions and health outcomes, as well as the relation between health outcomes and money. . . . " Outcomes management emphasizes reliance on standards and guidelines for selection of interventions; systematic measurement of the functioning and well-being of patients, particularly quality-of-life variables, along with disease-specific clinical outcomes; pooling of clinical and outcome data on a massive scale; and dissemination of results relevant to the needs of each group of information consumers. As a logical extension, payors might use such information to drive the health care system toward more efficacious selection of interventions by financial incentives that would reward the use of well demonstrated, efficacious interventions. Such information about quality of care from an outcomes perspective could also be used for utilization review purposes, to determine the relative marginal benefit of different interventions or of the same intervention at different levels of care for specific clinical problems, i.e., whether the patient can not only improve but do so less expensively.

All of the above approaches and combinations of them are used, explicitly and otherwise, as definers of quality; no single component dominates. When developing or assessing any system of quality assurance, it is important to clearly understand the definition of quality that is used. It is likely that a comprehensive system of quality assurance will incorporate elements of several of the above definitions.

Constraints on the Development of Quality Assurance Systems

Organizing and maintaining a good system to assure quality of care are limited by a number of formidable constraints. Not the least of these is the consensus required. There must be consensus about the definition of quality to be adopted. To the extent that adherence to certain standards of care is one approach to be pursued, there must be at least minimal consensus about the content of these standards. Because of rapid changes in knowledge and legitimate variations in practice style, this type of consensus can be difficult to achieve. Differences in the professional leadership structure of particular clinical specialties contribute to the problem. More autocratically controlled specialties may have less variance; newer specialties with multiple schools of thought may have more. Differences also exist with regard to the amount of scientifically validated knowledge available to particular specialties. Groups that lack common domain assumptions about which factors are important to a process may disregard scientifically validated findings from another group. While the belief is that some specialties, psychiatry for example, may have less consensus about standards of practice than do others, actual measures of consensus dispersion in medical specialties are lacking.

Another constraint is the dissociation of quality practices from desired outcomes of care. Systems that emphasize adherence to good practices, however defined, may not examine the effects of such practices on outcomes. In malpractice hearings, practitioners are not expected to achieve good outcomes, only to perform standard practice. Quality assurance systems that focus on quality through promoting adherence to well established procedures or at least avoidance of substandard ones may overlook the outcome component of quality. But even if outcome is included, measuring it in anything more than a rudimentary fashion is far beyond the resources of many health care systems.

Limited resources and time are also a problem. Physicians and others involved in health care are busy people, preoccupied with the delivery of health care. Even those organizations with full-time dedicated quality-assurance staffs have to deal with issues of limited resources and time. Any model that relies on labor intensive quality assurance activities, such as one in which there is some form of "looking over the shoulder" of each practitioner on every case, is extremely expensive and risks the problem of very marginal returns. Even heavily staffed quality assurance programs cannot address all possible quality issues. The need to focus on selected ones is an obviously limiting factor.

Practical systems of quality assurance also require efficient surveillance mechanisms. Direct observation of clinical practice, therefore, truly looking over the shoulder in vivo, gives way to proxies of actual practice. This usually takes the form of chart review rather than direct observation of practice. Inevitably, some information is lost, since chart review is based on selective and biased observations. Charting practices that conceal or misrepresent technical errors can further limit accurate surveillance.

Another extremely important constraint on the implementation of a good quality assurance system is related to conflicts over professional autonomy. Limited as they may be, the technologies for assessing quality of care are further developed than are techniques for assuring quality by modifying practitioner behavior. Practitioners who believe in the freedom to make clinical decisions within the limits of legality tend to resist efforts to alter their behavior to conform with standards imposed by others. Some (Eddy, 1990) resist establishing any rules of practice, even rules set by themselves, apparently in the belief that practice should be a matter of individual conscience or intuitive choice. Others may be less principled and simply not pay attention to the findings of quality assessment, perhaps out of disinterest or disagreement with it. In any event, converting quality assessment findings into new behavior by clinicians is often problematic.

Finally, constraints can be imposed by the type of quality assurance strategy adopted. Berwick (1989) has discussed the negative, self-defeating aspects of traditional "policing" systems. Such systems are at risk of inducing staff to conceal mistakes rather than seek methods to prevent or correct them. This is particularly true of retrospective quality assessment methods and quality assurance systems that do not permit those being assessed to participate in setting the standards. Theoretical and practical innovations in quality assurance technology in industry have led to the proposal that "continuous improvement" models of quality assurance, involving staff participation, be adopted in health care (Laffel, 1989). Such systems reward employees for detecting quality problems and for proposing practical solutions. Whether such methods can result in superior performance in health care remains to be seen.

Quality Assurance Approaches and Reviews

Efforts to deal with the problem of quality care, however defined, include quality assessment and assurance activities. Quality assessment refers to activities designed to ascertain the extent to which actual clinical practices conform to specified standards. It is an attempt to measure "how well we're doing." Quality assurance (QA) refers to activities designed to prevent and/or correct quality problems. In health care organizations, it is inherently a political process, for it requires systems intended to alter the behavior of practitioners and employees. Unless the organizational climate is favorable, making progress on QA is no small matter.

Several types of organizations have attempted to construct systems for quality assessment and assurance. These include organized medical/ professional groups, hospitals, and insurance carriers (Fauman, 1989). The earliest attempts to promote quality in patient care occurred in medical organizations such as the American College of Surgeons. The typical approach amounted to exhortations, education and self-monitoring. Despite the traditional belief in the value of peer review, for example, the early methods did not generally include looking over the shoulder of one's colleagues. Thinking back each day about cases, to consider how one might have done better represented the prevailing view.

Hospitals became involved in quality assurance essentially because of Joint Commission on Accreditation of Healthcare requirements and risk management concerns. Liability and dangers could be prevented or limited through QA programs, particularly because hospitals were deemed responsible for substandard care by medical staff members. Hospital QA has taken a variety of forms, typically relying on screening for poor quality care and attempting to correct aberrant practice patterns through practitioner education. Some hospitals have added retrospective chart review of individual cases, chart audits of specific problems (Performance Evaluation Procedure Audits), and problem identification through occurrence screening approaches, as well as systematic monitoring and evaluation of specific practices.

The Joint Commission on Accreditation of Healthcare Organizations (JCAHO, 1989) requires that accredited hospitals adhere to a 10-step monitoring and evaluation plan to focus on high-priority items. The process is composed of the following steps:

1. Assign responsibility for monitoring and evaluation activities;
2. Delineate the scope of care provided by the organization;
3. Identify the most important aspects of care provided by the organization;
4. Identify indicators (and appropriate clinical criteria) for monitoring the important aspects of care;
5. Establish thresholds (levels, patterns, trends) for the indicators that trigger evaluation of the care;
6. Monitor the important aspects of care by collecting and organizing the data for each indicator;
7. Evaluate care when thresholds are reached in order to identify either problems or opportunities to improve care;

8. Take actions to improve care or to correct identified problems;
9. Assess the effectiveness of the actions and document the improvement; and
10. Communicate the results of the monitoring and evaluation process to relevant individuals, departments, or services and to the organization's entire quality assurance program.

Hospital quality assurance systems often experience difficulty converting quality assessment into quality assurance. Medical disciplinary actions, for example, depend on the ability of the medical staff leadership to overcome the protectionism so characteristic of self-regulating organizations and on the hospital administration's commitment to improving the quality of care. Hospitals that have considered themselves to be successful in doing so have identified some of the factors that seem to help. Smith (1979) describes several:

1. A multidisciplinary, administrative, risk management steering committee "that provides guidance and resources for development of quality assurance standards and risk management procedures";
2. A quality assurance committee composed of physicians, the chair of the board of directors, the president, an attorney member of the board, and additional board members;
3. Routine physician profiles and medical audits;
4. Commitment and actual participation by the corporation president;
5. Medical executive committee assignment of responsibility to departmental committees for reviewing professional practices to reduce mortality and morbidity and improve patient care;
6. A patient education program guided by physicians to improve patient communication and understanding of procedures;
7. A continuing medical education program, driven by adverse findings of the medical audit committee and designed to remedy deficiencies; and
8. Early involvement of risk management staff in reported incidents.

Der Yuen (1986) describes a successful hospital departmental risk management committee, composed of department members, other specialty members, the department chief and the department medical director. Objective hearings are held on reports of alleged physician impairment, flagrant errors in clinical practice, or patterns of poor care. Educational efforts are applied to minor problems. More serious ones result in hearings before the committee, followed by a report to the medical executive committee, and possibly resulting in immediate suspension or restriction of privileges. "Without the whole-hearted support of the hospital executive committee, chief of staff, and administration, the existence and function of the risk management committee would not be possible" (Der Yuen, 1986).

Because of congressional concern that insurance carriers were inattentive to issues of medical necessity for hospital admissions, Medicare legislation required the development of Professional Standards Review Organizations (PSRO), subsequently renamed Professional Review Organizations (PRO). These were the first free-standing utilization review organizations, responsible for reviewing care for medical necessity. They were also charged with assuring quality of care, but there was no specific definition of quality nor a specific mandate to fulfill. Their activities were limited to the identification of "gross and flagrant" violations of standards of care. Only in the last few years did they engage in problem-focused medical audits for quality of care problems.

Some of the current remedies for quality-of-care problems in the Medicare program use sanctions such as financial penalties and exclusion from the program, but these only add to the already negative appeal of Medicare practice for many physicians (Lohr, 1990). Faced with discounted reimbursement rates, possible criminal penalties for billing errors, voluminous paperwork, and capricious interpretations of billing rules, the risks of additional penalties for violating undisclosed quality standards may be counterproductive for quality care if they influence good physicians to avoid Medicare practice altogether.

The interest of insurance companies and employers in cost containment has led to the development of utilization management companies. Typically, the care of individual patients is screened by non-medical personnel who refer cases that appear to fail screening criteria to medical peer reviewers (physician advisors) for further action. Attention to quality concerns ranges from little, in "pure" utilization review systems where the focus is on medical necessity, to considerable in managed care systems, particularly those tied to selected practitioner groups such as Preferred Provider Organizations (PPOs). These managed care systems typically allow practitioners wide latitude in clinical decision making. They rely on collegial persuasion by medical reviewers to influence practitioner behavior.

Quality assurance systems have generally used three types of information: structural, process, and outcome (Donebedian, 1980). "Structural" refers to the credentials and qualifications of staff as well as the adequacy of the organizational structure in which the care is provided. "Process" examines the adherence to standard rules of practice, emphasizing the "how and why" of practice. "Outcome" information includes the results of care, potentially including clinical improvement as well as adverse events. A comprehensive program includes all three. The relative emphasis on each as well as the timing (prospective, concurrent, and retrospective) are useful ways to characterize QA systems.

All QA systems are the result of trade-offs between a number of dimensions. These include:

1. Concurrent versus retrospective review
2. Outcome versus process review
3. Analysis of system processes versus practitioner performance
4. Internal versus external monitoring of quality
5. Reviews of acute hospital care versus reviews of lower levels of care
6. Review by peer consultation versus peer committee
7. Quality assessment versus quality assurance
8. Quality-enhancing versus quality-policing

Effective systems of QA should combine elements from both ends of each dimension. Because of limited time and resources, however, as well as differences in philosophy and purpose, the exact mix will vary.

Limitations on Current Outcome Indicator Approaches

For many reasons, hospital quality assurance systems have emphasized the retrospective review of adverse outcomes. Retrospective chart reviews are far less expensive than concurrent reviews. If not handled carefully, concurrent reviews can pose certain malpractice liability risks to peer reviewers for actions that might be construed as interventions in the care of patients. Many physicians prefer medical accountability systems that permit them wide latitude and independence at the time of service and leave professional review for later. And retrospective reviews are far less likely than concurrent reviews to precipitate direct confrontation between physicians.

Retrospective review is also attractive to hospital administrators. They are interested in reducing hospital exposure to liability and prefer processes that emphasize quality review of actual adverse events that could trigger a lawsuit. A very common approach to retrospective review consists of auditing samples of charts for the occurrence of pre-identified risk management concerns, i.e., adverse outcomes that place the hospital at legal risk. The hope is that identifying the sources of these adverse outcomes and implementing corrective efforts will prevent future recurrences. The increase in tort liability over the past decade or two has been closely linked to the rise of hospital interest in this type of review.

These predetermined adverse-outcome events are generally termed "outcome indicators." Specialty-specific indicators are created for each medical specialty in the hospital. The Hospital Association of New York State, for example, has proposed such outcome indicators for use by hospital members (Longo, 1989). For psychiatry, they are as follows:

Elopement
Hospital-incurred incident
Injury using restraints
Medication error
Staff noncompliance with hospital restraint policy
Suicide gesture/attempt while hospitalized
Unexpected drug reaction
Unplanned transfer to another acute care hospital

Although efficient for certain purposes, a system such as the above, is very limited if restricted to outcome indicators. First, this approach narrowly focuses on extreme adverse occurrences and does not examine issues of effectiveness. Second, while it draws attention to hospital-system as well as practitioner behavior, it may detract attention from practitioner deficiencies as the central focus. Third, risk management concerns tend to drive the choice of topics for examination. Although legitimate, this focuses attention on the prevention of adverse events rather than on the promotion of more effective care. Finally, this type of process is retrospective and reactive rather than concurrent and proactive. It emphasizes the prevention of future adverse occurrences rather than the correction of current risky situations. For those interested in the promotion of more effective care, such systems leave much to be desired.

Special Issues in Quality Assurance for Mental Health Services

There has long been a question about the extent to which mental health services are amenable to QA methods. At the center of this question is the feasibility of constructing consensually validated standards for quality mental health practice. The major differences between mental health professionals about the causes of emotional disturbance, the proliferation of schools of psychotherapy and overzealous practitioners with poorly substantiated and exaggerated claims of therapeutic potency, and limited knowledge of the biological processes underlying emotional disturbances have all contributed to skepticism about the ability to define, measure and assure the quality of mental health services.

Against this background is an emerging body of national practice standards for mental health services. The development of a scientifically validated body of knowledge regarding medical diagnostics and clinical psychopharmacology, a reliable psychiatric diagnostic typology (the American Psychiatric Association's DSM–III and DSM–III–R), and JCAHO standards for minimal documentation and evaluation of inpatient psychiatric problems have contributed to a core set of practice expectations for many common disorders. National organizations such as the American Psychiatric Association, the American Psychological Association, and the American Academy for Adolescent and Child Psychiatry have proposed guidelines for quality evaluation and treatment of diagnostic-specific disorders. The American Psychiatric Association developed peer review standards for psychiatric care in conjunction with its prior role as a national psychiatric peer review organization for CHAMPUS (health insurance for military dependents). Further, specialty and subspecialty board preparation and review courses have exposed national audiences of mental health practitioners to standards of care generated by leading academic research institutions. The argument that the mental health professions have no standards by which to judge quality is increasingly difficult to maintain.

Certain areas of mental health have far less well developed standards of care. There are still many diagnostic entities and problems that are poorly understood and researched, particularly those that show up in outpatient care, i.e., multiple personality and somatoform disorders. Standards for documentation of assessment and treatment of outpatient care are minimal compared to those for inpatient.

A more complex issue is whether standards of care can be operationalized. Quality assurance systems require measurable criteria of performance for quality assessment to occur. Once a quality standard has been established and criteria set, there must be unambiguous, measurable means for determining the extent to which the standard is being achieved. Are mental health standards such that they can be operationalized?

The DSM–III–R derives from operationalized diagnostic criteria sets constructed originally for clinical research purposes. Despite persisting controversy about their clinical validity, they have been well documented to be reliable, that is, capable of being predictably reproduced by different examiners. Some medical specialties are behind psychiatry in the development of operationalized criteria for common diagnostic entities that lack clear pathological tissue correlates, such as congestive heart failure, irritable bowel syndrome, and mitral valvular prolapse. No other medical specialty has developed a comparable, comprehensive, operationalized diagnostic typology as has psychiatry.

Psychopharmacological treatment is very amenable to operationalizing QA standards. Drug trials, as with lithium, can be assessed for adequacy in terms of blood concentration, duration of treatment, and presence of specific adverse effects. Appropriateness of drug selection can also be operationalized through identification of specific clinical syndromes that are associated with specific medication response, and subsequent measurement of adherence to guidelines for preferred medication choices.

To the extent that minimal assessment factors have been established as standards for mental health services, a simple categorical assessment for presence or absence can be used. To measure the validity of the clinical assessment is much more difficult, given the absence of well established pathophysiological and anatomic abnormalities that serve as "gold standards" in other medical specialties.

Because there are operationalized criteria for meeting standards of care, measurable indicators of mental health practice can be collected. At present, such measurements are generally limited to categorical, i.e., nominal judgments of whether a standard of behavior was met. An indicator of quality care in psychiatry, for example, might include the standard that potentially addictive medications such as benzodiazepines be withheld from known chemically dependent patients following drug detoxification. A practitioner's behavior either conforms to this standard or it does not. Crude though they may be statistically, such indicators are amenable to quantitative assessment.

The development of tools to define and measure the outcomes of mental health treatment has made outcome analyses possible. In addition to the gross standards of mortality and flagrant adverse outcomes, validated, standardized mood and behavior rating scales such as the

Hamilton Depression Scale and the Brief Psychiatric Rating Scale permit pre- and post-treatment analysis of change in patient condition. A variety of new tools for measuring quality of life, such as the Sickness Impact Profile and the Index of Well-being (Ellwood, 1988), promise even better assessment tools.

Psychotherapy research has begun the task of efficacy investigations. One interesting study by Smith and Associates attempting to estimate the overall efficacy of psychotherapy per se, found through a meta-analysis of 475 controlled studies that the average individual in psychotherapy fared better at the end of treatment than 80% of control subjects (Karasu, 1989). More sophisticated studies, attempting to measure the magnitude of the effects of psychotherapy, need to be completed. Studies examining the relative impact of psychotherapy on typical outcome indicators seen in hospital-based quality assurance also need to be performed.

Peer review of mental health care is possible and is being done. The nagging question remains, however, of whether it has any beneficial impact. The quality monitoring literature describes experiments in criteria-based analysis of inpatient psychiatric care (Edelstien, 1976), psychotherapy patients (Sarnat, 1979), prescribing of psychotropics in a community mental health center (Diamond, 1976), residential treatment of adolescents (Price, 1988), and treatment of long-term, difficult patients (Luft and Newman, 1988). The Luft and Newman study used a randomized, blinded comparison of the impact of peer review on high-risk patients, and showed no difference in outcome or service utilization. While the study's methodological adequacy may be questionable, the point is that quality assurance methods in mental health should be as subject to outcome analysis as are treatment methods.

Managed Mental Health Services

The hallmark of managed mental health services has been the transition from a traditional model based on a dyadic relationship between practitioner and patient to a triadic relationship between practitioner, patient, and a third party in the role of monitor. Perceived marked variations in utilization and in the quality of providers have led to the development of systems for data collecting, monitoring, critical review, and negotiated interventions in the service of promoting cost-effective, high-quality care.

Managed care and utilization review are not the same, despite the frequency with which the terms are used synonymously. Utilization review focuses on third-party determination of the medical necessity for treatment at a particular level of care or for a particular procedural intervention; in purest form, it is either a ratification or a veto of a treatment plan proposed by the practitioner. Managed care, however, strives to promote quality-enhanced care through arrangements that bring optimal clinical care to patients. Managed care involves case managers in diagnostic formulation, treatment planning, and critical analysis of therapeutic efforts. Managed care also maintains an enhanced longitudinal involvement in the patient's treatment needs, transcending specific episodes of illness, specific providers, and specific facilities.

A managed care system may promote a change in providers as well as in treatment plans where quality care does not seem to be forthcoming. In the purer models, a treating practitioner could become the technician who implements therapy in accordance with the case manager's assessment of the patient's treatment needs and who could be replaced if those needs are not being met. The core task of the case manager in a managed care system is to insure that the patient's care needs are being met— preferably *well* met—as opposed to the utilization reviewer's narrower duty to ensure that proposed treatment is medically necessary and reasonable.

In view of the wide variation in style and quality of mental health practitioners, managed mental health has attracted tremendous interest as a possible means to promoting effective care. A not infrequent observation of utilization reviewers is "the patient's condition is sufficiently severe to warrant inpatient treatment, but the type of diagnostic evaluation or treatment is inadequate to correct the problem." The organizational problem is that the patient *needs* treatment but the practitioner is providing the wrong kind. This is not a problem of over- or underutilization but of dysfunctional, ineffective, or inefficient care. The challenge in managed mental health is to insure that patients get better by receiving effective, high-quality care and that health benefits are not wasted on dysfunctional or unnecessary care.

Quality issues encompass two major areas in managed mental health systems. Broadly drawn, these include quality issues related to provider behavior and case manager behavior. A provider behavior might be misdiagnosis or failure to treat. Case manager behavior would include a premature denial of certification for extended inpatient care.

Managed mental health systems can operate in a variety of economic environments. When they are in the open, fee-for-service market, they can perform an important utilization review function by preventing overutilization. When they are in prepaid or fixed reimbursement environments, are at-risk and can profit from underservice, such arrangements can evoke conflicts of interests. How can an effective quality monitoring system be institutionalized in a system where there are financial incentives to underutilize?

There are several possible constraints on underservice in managed mental health systems. Practitioners can serve as patient advocates, particularly when they gain nothing from underservice. In such situations, they can argue with the case managers for the clinical benefits of longer or more resource-intensive service. When case management decisions are made prior to assignment of a clinical provider, as in some systems, responsibility for patient advocacy at the time of initial treatment planning becomes unclear. Sometimes external political forces such as unions or other beneficiary representatives function as patient advocates, unfortunately often without adequate clinical background.

Standards for managed mental health have become politicized in a number of states, where legislatures have mandated minimal criteria for utilization review organizations (Ryan, 1989). This legislation has addressed such issues as the credentials of front-line reviewers, requirements for physician determination of final certification decisions, requirements for identification of physician reviewers, and disclosure of screening criteria. Model standards for managed health care, let alone for managed mental health, have yet to appear. The strong interest in this is likely to lead to greater regulation in the future.

Virtually all managed mental health systems use screening criteria to determine medical necessity for acute hospital and other levels of care. Similar screening criteria for minimal standards of quality have not appeared. Some systems have tried to enter "the back door" of quality review by denying certification for care that does not meet minimal "intensity of service" criteria for hospital treatment. Such criteria are usually thought of as medical necessity rather than quality of care criteria. At some point, however, managed mental health systems will have to consider whether care should be subject to sanctions because it fails to meet quality criteria. Most managed care systems with a utilization review perspective stop short of responding to care that is not a "gross and flagrant" violation.

Just as standards and criteria to assess the quality of patient care are both possible and desirable, they should be developed for case management as well. Is the managed care program sufficiently knowledgeable of the patient's problems that require treatment? Does it critically evaluate the accuracy of the clinician's diagnoses? Does it assure that the proposed treatment plan logically corresponds to the stated diagnoses? Is an adequate course of treatment provided? Are adverse effects of treatment properly managed? Are rational changes made in the treatment plan if it appears that treatment is failing? Are new problems addressed that appear in the course of treatment? Is an adequate aftercare plan developed? Does the case manager identify opportunities for improved assessment and treatment? Does the case manager influence changes in treatment by appropriate interventions? All of these and other questions can form the basis for formulating standards, specific criteria, and indicators.

What role can managed care systems play in monitoring the quality of the provider network? Case managed systems rapidly become aware of wide variations in the quality of patient care among different providers, including individual practitioners and facilities. There are opportunities for case management intervention here, ranging from identification and management of consistently aberrant providers to the development of high-quality provider networks. Perhaps the greatest opportunities for managed mental health systems lie in the development of superior quality provider groups, going beyond screening for "gross and flagrant" violations of quality standards.

It is in everyone's interest to devise effective systems of internal quality assurance. The only legitimate justification for the existence of managed care systems has to do with whether they can provide superior, less costly, care compared to the traditional system. A well-designed and well-functioning internal QA system can help bring this about.

An External Quality Monitoring Program

Are at-risk managed mental health systems able to avoid underutilization and poor quality service? Can they develop well-functioning quality assurance systems? Or are their incentives and conflicts of interest too great for objective self-examination and self-regulation?

One useful attempt to answer these questions may be through an *external* quality monitoring process that screens cases for possible quality problems, as a means to identify possible underutilization and other concerns. There have been several such projects in which payors contract with outside experts to review the work of the managed mental health firm. Generally, the reviewers judge the quality of patient care in accordance with national standards of practice incorporated into generic and sometimes diagnosis-specific screening criteria. Typically, a statistically adequate sample of patient cases is reviewed by experienced clinicians. In larger studies, cases that fail screening criteria for quality care as applied by nurse reviewers are subsequently referred to senior psychiatrists and psychologists for peer review.

Based on these judgments, a quantitative analysis of problematic practices identifies high prevalence problems. Findings can be stratified in accordance with peer reviewer judgments about the severity of the quality problems. The reviews can include both patient care and case management decisions. Premature discharge from the hospital, for example, can be ascribed to the attending physician, to the case manager as a representative of the managed mental health firm, or to both.

Information gathered by the external monitor is made available to the payor, the providers and the managed mental health firm's internal quality assurance system. For those few firms with an internal system, comparison of the external monitor's findings with those of the internal system can reveal significant inconsistencies and can help improve the internal system.

Where is Quality Assurance in Managed Mental Health Going?

The potential for underservice in managed mental health is great enough to consider the use of external quality monitoring systems, at least in part because of the possibility that internal quality monitoring activities can be subverted to the interests of the managed mental health firm. Although the combination of internal and external quality monitors would seem to offer the best of both worlds, the burden of proof is on at-risk managed mental health systems to demonstrate whether any internal systems can really be effective. Independent quality monitoring systems can be more objective due to their greater distance from economic incentives for underutilization. For those managed mental health systems not at risk, the need for routine external quality monitoring is probably desirable but less compelling. Experience from periodic external quality audits should provide more information on this.

A difficult issue is how to convert quality assessment into quality assurance, how to alter the behavior of case managers and providers, when an external quality monitor has no direct authority over them. Resistance to criticism and to change can result in quality recommendations being ignored. To help with this problem, there needs to be a perception by the managed mental health system and the payor client that an external quality monitor can make a valuable contribution to the effectiveness of these systems and to the integrity of patient care. Systems that reject or ignore the findings of external review because they seem threatening risk long-term corruption. External quality monitors can help by keeping a focus on quality issues and by promoting patient advocacy. They can also help by promoting the goals of the managed mental health organization, improving performance, enhancing patient satisfaction, and positioning the organization more favorably in a competitive market. The added cost of external quality monitors is probably most justifiable to the degree that strong economic incentives may encourage underutilization.

External quality assurance monitors can be useful to case managers who may be sensitive to quality issues in an individual case, but may not necessarily track the quality performance of providers across cases and time. They can also be useful to those who contract with managed mental health systems by providing objective information on how the system is performing. By providing an objective information base for building a high-quality provider network through identifying superior practitioners they can also help both the managed care vendor and client.

An important lens through which to judge a managed mental health system has to do with whether it promotes more efficacious and efficient care as well as screening for substandard care. The concept that managed care is best done by "cutting out the fat" is somewhat hollow. Once the "fat" is cut out, there can be a lingering sense that the patient has still not been substantially helped. The goal should be to efficiently pull together interventions likely to actually help. To do so requires the introduction of high standards of quality and state-of-the-art knowledge. At present, these may be most easily available through external quality monitor systems.

Because external quality monitors add costs to a managed mental health system, it may make sense to have them paid by corporate clients and other purchasers of these systems. To minimize such costs, there is a need to learn how to do external quality monitoring efficiently. The technology is still in its infancy, and attempts to find better techniques should be encouraged.

THE FUTURE

Where should QA in managed mental health go? Given the early stage of development for QA in the managed mental health environment, there are many unanswered questions and much work to be done. There are several directions that appear to be promising.

1. Because they offer substantial opportunities for improvements in the quality of managed care, external quality monitoring should be considered seriously.

2. Systems of internal quality monitoring with diligent and responsive clinical supervision for case managers should be required in all managed mental health systems.

3. Managed mental health systems should develop somewhat different case management criteria than those used in conventional utilization review. In addition to the usual admission and continuing care criteria for acute hospital care, multiple levels of care criteria should be developed, taking into consideration a spectrum of alternate mental health services.

4. To help reduce the potential for underutilization, criteria for discharge from each level of care or for transfer to a higher level of care should be developed. Admission/continuing-care criteria have helped to reduce the subjectivity of utilization decisions; greater consensus on terminating care, transferring it to either a lower or higher level is needed.

5. Quality assurance systems should continue to develop better criteria for typical patterns of high quality care for specific problems. This is part of a process for arriving at consensually validated standards of high quality care. QA as a means to promote better care should replace such older concepts of quality assurance as identifying and weeding out flagrant examples of substandard care. As indicators of efficacy are developed, it should be possible to compare the quality of managed mental health systems across competitors.

6. Better indicators of efficacy of outcomes should be developed as well as indicators of adverse outcomes. These would rest on the answers to such questions as: What are the best ways to know if patients improve with treatment? Will managed mental health systems require providers to collect measures of the condition of the patient before and after treatment? Which measures should be

employed? Will systematic comparison of different treatment interventions be undertaken to test beliefs about which treatments and which levels of care really work?

7. Process quality studies should be continued to analyze practice patterns for comparison with professional rules of practice. They should not be abandoned in favor of outcome studies as has been the case in hospital QA systems.

8. Standards of practice should be developed for case managers. Some of the areas that should be included have been cited above. One of the important ones has to do with the extent to which they function as patient advocates.

Finally, a national data bank should be established for the collection, analysis, and dissemination of quality assessment findings in mental health, as Ellwood (1988) has suggested for all medical specialties. Little is known about variations in regional practice or about the extent of deviation from national standards. Even though it is in the competitive nature of things for managed mental health systems to develop proprietary information about quality assurance and be reluctant to share it, the ultimate goal is for all patients to benefit from what is learned.

REFERENCES

Berwick, D.N.: Continuous improvement as an ideal in health care. *New England Journal of Medicine, 320:*53–56, 1989.

Der Yuen, D.: A large community hospital's experience with an obstetrics-gynecology risk management committee. *Am J Obstet Gynecol, 154:*1206, 1986.

Diamond, H., Tislow, R., Snyder, T. Jr, et al: Peer review of prescribing patterns in a CMHC. *Am J Psychiatry, 133:*697, 1976.

Donabedian, A.: Explorations in Quality Assessment and Monitoring Vol. I, *The Definition of Quality and Approaches to Its Assessment.* Ann Arbor, Michigan, Health Administration Press, 1980.

Eddy, D.M.: The challenge. *JAMA, 263:*287, 1990.

Edelstien, M.G.: Psychiatric peer review: A working model. *Hosp Community Psychiatry, 27:*656, 1976.

Ellwood, P.A.: Outcomes management: A technology of patient experience. *New England Journal of Medicine, 318:*1549, 1988.

Fauman, M.A.: Quality assurance monitoring in psychiatry. *Am J Psychiatry, 146:*1121, 1989.

Joint Commission on Accreditation of Healthcare Organizations: *1990 Accreditation Manual for Hospitals.* Chicago, JCAHO, 1989.

Karasu, T.B.: New frontiers in psychotherapy. *J Clin Psychiatry, 50:*46, 1989.

Laffel, G., Blumenthal, D.: The case for using industrial quality management science in health care organizations. *JAMA, 262:*2869, 1989.

Lang, D.A.: The case for consultation. *Healthcare Executive,* 2:40, 1987.

Lohr, K.N., Schroeder, S.A.: A strategy for quality assurance in Medicare. *New England Journal of Medicine, 322:*707, 1990.

Longo, D.R., Ciccone, K.R., Lord, J.T.: *Integrated Quality Assessment: A Model for Concurrent Review.* American Hospital Publishing, 1989.

Luft, L.L., Newman, D.E.: Peninsula Hospital community mental health center quality assurance system. In Stricker, G., Rodriguez, A.R. (Eds.): *Handbook of Quality Assurance in Mental Health.* New York, Plenum, 1988.

MacKenzie, K.R.: Recent developments in brief psychotherapy. *Hosp Community Psychiatry, 39:*742, 1988.

Price, S.B., Greenwood, S.K.: Using treatment plans for quality assurance monitoring in a residential center. *QRB, 14:*266, 1988.

Ryan, P.: State regulation of utilization review organizations. CEO Forecast, memo, December 1, 1989.

Sarnat, J.E., Whitaker, L.C. and Arnstein, R.L.: Psychotherapy quality assessment. *J Am Coll Health, 28:*131, 1979.

Smith, J.R., Louks, J.L. and Petrocine, W.J.: The use of a multidisciplinary committee to manage the risk of suicide in a VA domiciliary. *QRB,* 211, 1986.

Smith, N.G.: A systemwide quality assurance/risk management program. *The Hospital Medical Staff, 8:*40, 1979.

Chapter 11

MANAGED MENTAL HEALTH: CLINICAL MYTHS AND IMPERATIVES

H. G. Whittington

The economic imperatives of managed care have been more visible than its ethical rectitude and clinical correctness. This is particularly true in mental health and substance abuse services, where technology assessment has been so little utilized, and many providers have found it profitable to stick to the canard that "we don't know what works."

Since the community mental health center program fueled systems research in its mandated program evaluation efforts, research on the outcome of mental health services related to locus, intensity, duration, and type of treatment intervention has grown steadily in this country. The research shows, beyond question, that much of the "treatment" afforded in the United States today is not that which is likely to be most cost-beneficial to the consumer, just as the profit and loss statements of the providers show that it is most cost-beneficial to them!

What the scientific literature does show includes the following:

1. A wide variety of biopsychosocial interventions are of proven effectiveness;
2. There is no general superiority of prolonged and expensive interventions over brief, more affordable ones;
3. Hospitalization is the least effective and most dangerous intervention, in spite of its popularity;
4. Biological treatments, where appropriate, are less expensive and equally effective, when used alone or in conjunction with briefer psychosocial therapy, as compared with exclusively psychosocial interventions;
5. It is possible to manage services and allocate resources to allow for greater penetration of the population-at-risk, at lesser cost, and with superior outcome than an unmanaged fee-for-service system can achieve;

6. Certain fixed ideas about managing the utilization of mental health and substance abuse programs are without foundation, and are counter-productive; and

7. Scientifically-based methods to manage care to an optimal (from a cost-benefit perspective) intensity and level do exist.

Before going on to the positives, it is useful to examine certain false assumptions that tend to cloud or distort our vision.

MYTHS THAT WILL NOT DIE

Decisions about resource allocation are based on ideas, the currency of human endeavors. As in other forms of commerce, the genuine must be separated from the counterfeit, if we are to avoid bankruptcy. In managed care, ideas must be tested against experience, utilizing the scientific method. If we do so, we find that many of the commandments of our enterprise are false, weakening the foundation of our systems. Some of these spurious but powerful notions are as follows:

Myth 1: Controlling physician behavior is simple: leave a trail of money and doctors will follow you anywhere.

There is no question that economic incentives influence human behavior, but not as simply and predictably as one might expect. A recent study (Hillman, 1989) showed that even with a complex analysis that included not only incentive and HMO-descriptive variables, but also market-area variables, only 40% of the variation in hospitalization rates could be accounted for. If only the physician reimbursement system is considered, only 15% of the variation in hospitalization rates is explained. Clearly, physicians are still, even in salaried and capitated systems, making decisions involving variables other than financial ones. And the study further showed that certain widely utilized mechanisms—such as withholding accounts, or bonuses based on productivity—were not important in predicting hospitalization rates.

Myth 2: Mental health and substance abuse services should account for less than 10% of managed care expenditures.

As levels approach and exceed 10%, a cry of alarm goes up about abusive overutilization, and more restrictive benefits and/or limitations on access are called for. But who really knows how much is "enough"?

And, if the supply of services is inadequate to meet the real need, what are the consequences for the managed care system?

Epidemiologic studies, spanning more than two decades, show a surprising constancy in estimates of prevalence of psychiatric and substance abuse disorders. Most recently, the National Institute of Mental Health (NIMH) Epidemiological Catchment Area program produced a stream of data about the lifetime prevalence and incidence of psychiatric disorders. In a study of lifetime prevalence (Robins et al, 1984), totals ranged from 25.7% for women in St. Louis to 39.6% for men in Baltimore. While college-educated, non-black, and suburban/small town/rural had slightly lower rates, and the young (25–44) the highest, no segment of the population was immune. In a six-month period, prevalence rates varied from a low of 11.5% in St. Louis to 13.2% in New Haven, with Baltimore at 12.5% (Myers et al, 1984). When we add these data to those suggesting an increase in prevalence in certain disorders (such as depression, particularly among the young, and cocaine addiction), it is clear that projections governing the staffing and financing of mental health and substance abuse services have been egregiously inadequate and shortsighted.

Study after study (Diehr et al., 1985; Shemo, 1986; Borus et al., 1985; McFarland et al., 1985; Mumford et al., 1984) has clearly shown that untreated or inadequately treated, psychiatrically ill or substance-abusing members consume an inordinate volume of general medical services. With proper treatment, the costs of this unnecessary, ineffective, and inappropriate medical treatment are significantly reduced.

Myth 3: Adverse selection will occur if good mental health benefits are offered.

Restriction of mental health benefits is rationalized as necessary because if good benefits are available, all the emotionally unstable people in town will seek care, there will be very high utilization and costs will skyrocket. Research does not support these alarmist beliefs (McGuire and Fairbank, 1988; Wells et al., 1986). Those in a fee-for-service plan and an HMO are equally likely to utilize services in a year; the costs are lower in an HMO due partly to fewer visits, but mainly to the use of psychiatric social workers rather than psychiatrists and psychologists, and because of reliance on group therapy. Data from the Rand Health Insurance Study (Wells, 1986) showed "no evidence of appreciable or significant adverse selection into or out of the prepaid group practice."

Myth 4: Psychotherapy is a moral hazard.

The alternative rationalization for the limitation of mental health benefits, particularly outpatient psychotherapy, is that individuals not in need of any treatment will somehow be lured (presumably by their own greed or lack of moral fiber) into utilizing psychotherapy simply because it is a covered benefit; or, once in needed therapy, will linger too long because of motivations unrelated to need for treatment of bonafide illness. Here, the prejudice against women, long seen as the helpless prey and chief source of income of psychotherapists, is most evident. (Although sexism permeates public and private policy at every level, it is no accident that alcoholism, seen as a man's disease, has had the most liberal benefits mandated by state legislatures; while drug abuse attributed to minorities and adolescents, and non-psychotic disorders requiring outpatient psychotherapy, the domain of the "bored housewife," have received short-shrift.)

The reality is that most patients do not linger long in psychotherapy (Blackwell et al., 1988), even in a clinic oriented toward long-term psychotherapy (Howard et al., 1989). Analysis of data from the National Medical Care Utilization and Expenditure Survey showed that one-third of the long-stay patients (the 9.4% who made 25 or more outpatient visits) were highly disabled and had multiple medical disorders (Taube et al., 1988). A careful analysis of the rationalizations justifying exclusion of outpatient psychotherapy benefits (Goldman and Taube, 1988) concludes, "A policy that presents few financial barriers to initiating treatment but limits excessive use could control costs responsibly and increase the access to care for the large proportion of the population who have mental disorders but do not use any mental health services. . . . A policy that encourages necessary use and controls moral hazard satisfies insurance principles and promotes public health."

But does the availability of services increase the number of patients who will avail themselves of psychiatric treatment? The answer here probably lies in the results of an "experiment of nature"—the market expansion through advertising that the proprietary chains of psychiatric hospitals have undertaken, with increasing investment in television time. Two markets have proven to be expandable; that for inpatient treatment of adolescent behavior problems, and for inpatient treatment of substance abuse. These psychiatric hospitals have been relatively unsuccessful, in primary markets with existing services, in increasing inpatient utilization by adult psychiatric patients. It is noteworthy that both of the two groups most responsive—adolescents and substance abusers—to some extent have diminished freedom of choice and are a burden on other people. Both populations, rightly or wrongly, are treated almost exclusively by psychosocial techniques, with no reliance on biologically-based treatment modalities. And, for both groups, psychiatrists have much less involvement as gatekeepers and directors of treatment. Admittedly, the proprietary chains have not pushed their marketing of outpatient services, for obvious reasons; but there is reason to believe, at present, that advertising can greatly increase the utilization of ambulatory services.

Another experiment of nature is the Canadian National Health System. Barer (1989) writes, "There is no evidence that user fees deter unnecessary use and lower health care costs." Coupled with the universal coverage in Canada, and legislation in 1987 that essentially abolished user fees, the lack of an expansion in the outpatient mental health market suggests that fears that the "worried well," not really in need of mental health treatment, would access outpatient psychotherapy, is probably unfounded.

Admittedly, the data in the United States are somewhat contradictory. If extreme differentials in cost of outpatient psychotherapy exist, utilization of mental health providers does decrease when all or most of the cost is borne by the individual. But the data do not tell us whether this is good or bad. Was unnecessary treatment avoided by financial disincentives? Or was necessary treatment simply forgone? What was the differential impact on general health status? Did patients simply consult general medical professionals, who submitted diagnoses and billings that were not reflective of the true mental status of the patient? Can we make treatment, including mental health care, so expensive that many people, no matter how great their need, cannot afford it? Certainly. Can we set up financial parameters so that those who do not "really need treatment" will not utilize resources? The answer to that question is much less clear.

Myth 5: Primary care physicians make good gatekeepers.

Not if we want patients to have needed psychiatric treatment! The longing of psychiatrists and other mental health professionals to be accepted by their more "scientific" medical brethren results in a romantic quest to educate them, to turn primary care physicians into sensitive case finders. But the achievement of that goal is no closer than it was 25 years ago. Both adult and pediatric physicians grossly under-identify psychiatric and substance abuse morbidity (Borus et al, 1988; Costello et al, 1988).

It is encouraging to see that physicians in managed care settings do eventually recognize this; but only after patients have been denied appropriate access during the early years of an HMO. In their first two years, only 22% of HMOs allow self-referral for mental health services, rising to 51% by 2–5 years of existence; and, if they are still around in 16 years, 80% allow self-referral (Shadle and Christianson, 1988). If only the learning curve could be steeper! And if only every HMO did not have to start from scratch, so that ontogeny recapitulates phylogeny.

Myth 6: More is better.

There is a strong belief that hospital treatment is better than outpatient treatment, long hospitalization must be better than short, and so on. These ideas have so much face validity that they are difficult to dispute.

Yet, a survey of published studies (Canton and Cralnick, 1987) refutes this notion. In uncontrolled studies of adult hospitalization, there is no difference in the re-hospitalization rate, related to duration of hospitalization, for five of the studies. Four of the studies showed no positive relationship between length of stay and effectiveness of role functioning, and one showed that the longer the hospitalization, the worse social role functioning was. Only one study showed a positive correlation between length of inpatient treatment and post-hospital functioning.

The literature is no less voluminous in the area of child and adolescent services, but less decisive. This is for a curious reason, however: most of the research has been done in the public sector, and the private hospitals now treating significant numbers of middle-class adolescents have contributed precious little to the outcome literature. A far-reaching literature survey (Melton, 1986) concludes, however, "every study that has compared the efficacy of treatment for clients randomly assigned to inpatient or alternative services has found the latter to be at least as effective (usually more effective)."

Myth 7: Managed care makes money by denying services.

As previously cited studies indicate (McGuire and Fairbanks, 1988; Wells et al., 1986), HMOs provide services to at least as many of the population-at-risk as fee-for-service systems do. More likely, over time, HMOs have a higher penetration than fee-for-service arrangements

(Manning et al., 1987). Claims paid data of at least one major managed care system (The Prudential), when compared with typical indemnity utilization, confirms that managed care offers service to more individuals; while in an unmanaged system, fewer people consume a larger share of resources, and many get no care at all. Cost savings in HMOs result from minimizing the use of inpatient confinement, the most costly component; increasing the utilization of day hospital and intensive outpatient treatment as alternatives to hospitalization; employing group modalities more extensively; and employing multi-disciplinary teams, with higher proportions of lower cost professionals.

Myth 8: Managed care results in poorer service outcomes.

This is really the key question—and not surprisingly, the one that is not entirely answered. There need to be large studies done of treatment outcomes in managed versus unmanaged settings. But, to the author's knowledge, no adequate research results have yet been published.

All of the major providers of managed care conduct patient satisfaction surveys on a regular basis. Some, such as Prudential, utilize an external survey firm to avoid bias. All report a high degree of patient satisfaction. Unfortunately, the fee-for-service system does not have comparable data.

The most frequently expressed concern is that utilization management efforts result in premature discharges from inpatient care, with poor results in consequence. One study of this in managed mental health has been done by National Medical Audit, and reported at the 1989 Annual Meeting of the American Psychiatric Association (Anderson, 1989). A national physician panel conducted blind reviews of 201 cases; there was no correlation between global ratings of quality of care and length of stay allowed.

Earlier research on health maintenance organizations demonstrated no differences in quality of care (Luft, 1980). However, subsequently, Luft (1988) was writing, "Unfortunately, this evidence is rather thin and, more importantly, the medical environment is changing in ways that make the available data increasingly irrelevant. . . . The HMO industry now has an incentive to focus on outcomes and health status measures to support their claims of quality."

Additionally, recent evidence (Wells, 1989) suggests that capitation payment systems may impede appropriate referral of psychiatric patients to specialized care. This, of course, has been a fear of mental health professionals for a long time, knowing that it is easy to disrupt help-seeking behavior in many psychiatric patients, who are vulnerable to rejection and prejudicial scapegoating.

Clearly, the evidence is not yet in on this vital issue. While in managed care, the cost-benefit ratio appears to be more favorable for the entire population-at-risk than in fee-for-service, this public health response does not soothe the superego of the patient-oriented mental health professional, for example, who necessarily and properly views the world one patient at a time.

Myth 9: The treatment of substance abuse requires a fixed length (usually 28 days) of inpatient treatment.

Rarely has a fixed belief had so little factual support, or been so fervently adhered to! As early as 1983, a report for the Office of Technology Assessment (Saxe, 1983), failed to demonstrate a general superiority of inpatient over alternative treatment settings, as measured by outcome. An update by the same author (Saxe, 1988) shows that the data are now even more compelling: hospital or residential treatment is neither a necessary nor sufficient treatment for most alcoholics. While the data base is smaller, the same appears to be true for other chemical dependencies.

Myth 10: Mental health is unmanageable.

This rationalization is the capstone, further justifying the management of mental health and substance abuse by benefit limits and exclusions. It is the classical "wooden leg game" a la Erik Berne: "If only I didn't have this wooden leg, I'd run in the marathon!"

Mental health and substance abuse services are easier to manage than general medical and surgical services: there are fewer diagnoses, fewer tests, fewer procedures, fewer rapid changes in technology. Denial of this is another manifestation of the general rejection of psychiatric patients and mental health professionals by the medical establishment. Unfortunately, with few exceptions (Langman-Dorwart, 1988; Goldstein et al., 1988) the utilization management in mental health systems is proprietary, a real impediment to good utilization research. On the occasions when mental professionals working in utilization management programs have an opportunity to discuss their work candidly, it is clear that there has been a high degree of convergence in the independently developing systems. There are no surprises, no secrets. Differences arise from cut-points (i.e., how suicidal do you have to be to merit inpatient treatment?), procedures (i.e., does a psychiatrist communicate with the treating physician before denial?), and quality of personnel, organization and supervision.

Myth 11: Most mental health treatment is discretionary; the patient is not really sick.

The belief is widespread among physicians that psychiatric treatment is equivalent to cosmetic surgery or dermatology, and hence not "medically necessary"—a neat rationalization for cutting benefits for mental health and substance abuse treatment to the bone.

Analysis of the Rand Medical Outcomes Data (Wells et al., 1989) covering 11,242 outpatients in three U.S. sites, shows that, "The poor functioning uniquely associated with depressive symptoms, with or without depressive disorder, was comparable with or worse than that uniquely associated with eight major chronic medical conditions." Who would dream of limiting benefits for these eight conditions—hypertension, diabetes, advanced coronary artery disease, angina, arthritis, or back, lung, and gastrointestinal disorders?

The implications are clear: "There is a gap between the research findings and the attitudes of some of the general public and unfortunately, at times, the medical profession. In some instances, depression is seen as a sign of moral or personal weakness rather than an illness worthy of medical attention. Changing attitudes of the public and of the general medical practitioners—should have a high priority for preventive programs as well as for clinicians, investigators, and policy makers" (Klerman, 1989).

People with panic attacks frequently present to primary care physicians with somatic complaints. About 1.5% of the population, at some time in their lives, experiences panic disorder; and panic attacks, which do not meet the diagnostic criteria fully, are two or three times as prevalent. New research, drawn from a random sample of 18,011 adults from five U.S. communities, shows that the risk of suicide is greatly elevated in this population. Twenty percent of the subjects with panic disorder had attempted suicide, as had 12% of those with panic attacks (Weissman, 1989). "A history of suicide attempts is one of the most powerful predictors of subsequent death by suicide. Of persons who make unsuccessful suicide attempts, approximately 1% commit suicide each year during the 10 years after the attempt" (Reich, 1989).

By age 45, approximately 20% of men with schizophrenia have committed suicide (Drake et al., 1985). When we add schizophrenia, panic disorders and attacks to the previously documented risk of suicide with depression, alcoholism, aging, chronic physical diseases, and personal losses, it is hard to trivialize psychiatric treatment, or to justify its exclusion from broad coverage.

The "realness" of mental illness is also shown in a study (Willard et al., 1983) focused on the management of suicide attempts among a psychiatric emergency room population; the outcome measure was death by suicide after discharge. The 5,284 psychiatric emergency room patients were followed-up for six months to seven years and yielded a suicide rate of 111.1 (per 100,000) patient years-at-risk, more than seven times the age- and sex-adjusted rates for the general population. While no patients had killed themselves immediately after an emergency room visit, "several had killed themselves without following through on a referral from the emergency room to another facility."

THE REALITIES OF MANAGED MENTAL HEALTH CARE

The Effectiveness Of Treatment

There is now a general recognition that sufficient outcome literature exists to support the clinical effectiveness of all of the major mental health treatment modalities. Therefore, we no longer have to deal with the issue, "Does treatment work?" but rather with the issue of, "What treatment works best for a particular condition?" A previously cited study (Caton and Cralnick, 1987), for example, supports the general usefulness of psychiatric hospitalization.

Psychopharmacology is widely recognized as an effective treatment for an increasing variety of conditions, currently including major depression, anxiety and phobic disorders, obsessive compulsive disorder, schizophrenia, Tourette's syndrome, organically-induced mental aberrations (such as partial, complex seizures), bipolar disorder, attention deficit disorder—and the list grows longer every year. The general experience in managed care systems is that those disorders having a specific and effective biological treatment do *not* generate excessive utilization demands on or costs to the system.

Problems *are* seen with those conditions for which there is not a generally accepted biological approach, where treatment is entirely psychosocial and administered by a multidisciplinary team, particularly if some element of coercion is being exerted against the patient (either legal, familial, or occupational), such as in adolescent and substance abuse programs. However, once this is said, there is substantial evidence that in almost all of these conditions, combining medication with psychosocial and behavioral therapies improves the outcome.

The general effectiveness of psychotherapy is now also clear. The introduction of meta-analytic techniques by Smith et al. (1980) laid the groundwork for a consensus that psychotherapy is a reasonably effective treatment method. The overall effect size, based on 475 studies in the literature between 1941 and 1976, was approximately 0.85; that is, a patient who is only better than 50% of the cohort prior to treatment, would be better off than 80% of the cohort after psychotherapy, if the rest remained untreated. The authors also conclude that if placebo therapy is omitted from the treated group, the effect size rises to 0.93. Another observation is that the more specific forms of treatment are more effective than generalized supportive techniques.

Alternatives To Hospitalization

Partial (day, evening and weekend) treatment programs have been in existence for over 30 years, and extensively researched both in the United States and Europe. A report by Schene and Gersons (1986) summarizes the many outcome studies that have been done over the last 15 years. The authors' summary is that, "The general conclusion is that partial hospital can be a reasonable alternative to inpatient as well as to outpatient treatment, taking into account factors such as symptomatology, cost, and family burden. Partial hospital seems in particular to enhance social functioning, which might be attributed to the fact that contact between the patient and environment is not disturbed by hospitalization."

Another recent article that reviews studies on the evaluation of partial hospitalization programs in North America and Europe, concludes that "The validity of the day hospital as an economical, effective treatment alternative for a substantial number of acutely ill patients is firmly established by well designed, large scale, controlled and replicated studies. Further research on the general validity of day hospitals would be superfluous" (Rose, 1987).

In looking more specifically at the use of partial hospitalization as an alternative to inpatient care, Pang (1985) concludes that, "Partial hospitalization can offer a viable alternative to inpatient hospitalization with less stigma and less family burden per patient. Such patients fare as well or better than inpatient counterparts."

Parker and Knoll (1990), while supporting the efficacy of partial hospitalization as a treatment modality, also point to a key impediment in increasing utilization. "It is our opinion that until more psychiatrists are trained in the use of partial hospitalization, more standardization of partial hospitalization takes place, and third-party payors economically direct patients and physicians toward partial hospitalization, the underutilization of this therapeutically and economically proven treatment modality will continue. The solution is simple; the implementation is complex."

Less Restrictive Treatment for Substance Abuse

As previously cited (Saxe, 1983, 1988), the data are compelling that intensive outpatient or partial hospitalization provide outcomes equal to those of inpatient or residential treatment for substance abuse. An article in the *New England Journal of Medicine* (Hayashida et al., 1989) concluded, "Outpatient medical detoxification is an effective, safe, and low cost treatment for patients with mild/moderate symptoms of alcohol withdrawal."

Faced with declines in utilization, inpatient facilities have been developing programs that are purported to be "dual diagnosis" units, thus justifying the use of inpatient treatment with this population. There are no good outcome studies of this population, however, and no professional consensus has developed as to the appropriate criteria for inpatient treatment.

Increasing emphasis is being placed on identifying subtypes of alcoholics and other substance abusers. This should make the outcome literature more sensitive (Nace, 1984) to differential treatment effects. The literature is generally moving toward more analysis of treatment alternatives to the traditional "12-step program," with the focus on outcome studies of behavioral approaches (Litman and Topham, 1983). Attempts to relate outcome to specific diagnostic categories, as well as to behavioral or demographic characteristics, also show some promise (Schuckit et al., 1986).

In summary, there is no evidence attesting to the general superiority of inpatient or residential treatment to outpatient or partial hospitalization approaches. The homogeneous quality of substance abuse programs in the United States, however, has deprived us, these last two decades, of good outcome studies that look at different approaches to treatment and use a more sophisticated typology of substance abuse. Much research needs to be done to really answer the central question: Which patients need inpatient treatment and rehabilitation, and which can benefit equally well from outpatient or partial hospitalization?

Brief Psychotherapy

The literature is clear in its support of the general effectiveness of briefer psychotherapeutic approaches. Horowitz et al. (1986) conclude that, "From all perspectives . . . major symptom relief occurred in the majority of patients, with less change in adaptive abilities." Another recent study of short-term dynamic psychotherapy, with a two year follow-up, indicated that 67% of the patients contacted after two years showed symptom relief. Another study reported that a five-year follow-up of these 39 original patients supported the conclusions of the original article (Husby et al., 1985).

In a survey article, MacKenzie (1988) identifies trends in therapeutic practice, with a shift to an interpersonal rather than intrapsychic focus of therapy. This has been accompanied by the development of more systematic techniques for defining the therapeutic focus, with increasing emphasis on brief psychotherapy, seen as a specific modality or set of techniques (rather than just a shorter version of long-term therapy).

As has been true for many years, the outcome studies of the benefit of psychotherapy for many "psychosomatic" or mind-body problems continue to be highly favorable. This certainly has implications for managed care systems, because of the offset value that results from a reduced utilization of medical services when such patients are treated effectively. Studies of such conditions as irritable bowel syndrome (Svedlund and Sjodin, 1985) and migraine headaches (Friedman and Taub, 1985), both of which have a great deal of outpatient office contact with general physicians, show significant and sustained improvement with brief psychotherapy.

Continuity of Care

Continuity of care is another principle that all practitioners support but rarely engage in. Yet, there can be no doubt of the clinical value of a system that promotes continuity within a managed care environment. A survey article by McKelvy (1988) presents a model for a continuum of care from inpatient to outpatient services on one campus, by combining the resources of a mental health program and a child social welfare agency.

Particular attention has been focused on the seriously disabled patient, when evaluating the positive effect of continuity of care (Santiago et al., 1985). Authors of this study, which utilized an integrated service approach, concluded that the experimental group showed substantive improvement in psychosocial functioning, although there were minimal differences in symptomatology and psychopathology.

Another study (Tessler, 1987) of a cohort of 112 clients, who were predominantly young white males, showed that at six months following discharge from a public mental health hospital, those with continuous care showed better adjustment to community living and a reduction of complaints from all sources. The total number of services recommended but not received showed the largest effect, with those individuals receiving continuous treatment being much more likely to follow through on recommended post hospital treatment.

In summary, the research literature has established that all of the major therapies, whether biological or psychosocial, will be of at least some benefit to most patients; this treatment can take place in a variety of settings; and there is no general advantage of inpatient, 24-hour a day treatment compared to less restrictive settings.

In consequence, a managed mental health approach would conclude that whenever possible, care should be provided on an outpatient basis, or in a day or evening treatment setting, and with pharmacological means if suitable for the diagnosis. Beyond that, a managed approach would, because of the outcome literature, favor psychosocial treatments that are brief rather than more prolonged, involve a family or a group approach, focus on intensive intervention at the time of crisis and follow the patient through the continuum of care until remission is firmly established. And, since relapse is often precipitated by social and environmental factors substantially external to the patient, treatment should extend into the social-surround, or be provided in a social setting that simulates the natural environment of the patient. In this way, treatment can prepare the patient to successfully cope with the psychonoxious influences that are likely to result in relapse, if the patient's adaptive capacity does not increase. Therefore, halfway houses, therapeutic foster care, and in-home family-centered child advocacy should all be part of the managed care continuum.

Crisis Intervention

Research supports the validity of the crisis intervention concept: helping individuals successfully manage or cope with life crises (that occur with predictable regularity in all of our lives) results over time in a diminution in the incidence of subsequent psychiatric morbidity and it can significantly reduce the inappropriate use of inpatient care. A study by Bengelsdorf and Alden (1987) found that crisis services in a psychiatric emergency room were able to prevent hospitalization in 70% of the crisis patients seen.

Raphael (1983) studied the effectiveness of preventive intervention in lowering post-bereavement morbidity in 200 widows. Those at risk for morbidity were selected and randomly assigned to experimental and control groups. The experimental groups received specific support for grief, and were encouraged to mourn during the first three months; whereas, no intervention was given to the control group. All were followed up 13 months later with a validated health questionnaire. The study showed that there was a significant decrease of morbidity in the intervention group as compared to the control group.

Other research has attempted to identify patient characteristics and therapeutic techniques that influence outcome. A survey of 67 patients (Bolvin et al., 1983) referred to an outpatient crisis intervention program, indicated that the best outcome was obtained with middle-aged, high socioeconomic status patients with a single, mild to moderately severe life stress. An eclectic therapeutic approach with non-specific therapeutic techniques that are positive, supportive, and forward-looking gave the best results.

The potential contribution that crisis intervention can make to ongoing practice in a managed care system is exemplified in a study of crisis intervention counseling in medical-surgical patients (Viney et al., 1985). This study examined the psychological reaction of 259 female and 130 male medical and surgical patients between the ages of 18 and 60 years. At time of discharge and at 12 month follow-up, women who received crisis intervention during their hospitalization showed psychological gains when compared with non-counseled women, expressing fewer feelings of helplessness and more of competence in the short term, and less anxiety and helplessness in the long term. While men showed some improvement in the short term, there were fewer demonstrated gains in the long term. Overall, patients receiving crisis intervention counseling showed less anxiety on discharge and fewer depressive feelings on follow-up.

To consider several of these aspects of the managed care clinical philosophy:

Family Therapy

Family therapy has been demonstrated to be a highly cost effective treatment modality and should be part of the managed mental health program. Recent studies have focused on brief family therapy (Fisher, 1988). A study of family therapy comparing outcomes after one year between families treated with six session time-limited therapy, 12 session time-limited therapy, or treated without time limits, showed no significant differences in outcome. The author concludes, "However, time limits did succeed in shortening treatment, without significantly reducing its effectiveness or the durability of outcome."

The value of family therapy in improving outcome of hospital-based treatment has also been substantiated. A study by Hass et al. (1988) showed that at the time of discharge, patients randomly assigned to inpatient family intervention showed improved outcomes, particularly in females with major affective disorder. The same authors reported, however, at six-month and 18-month follow-ups (Spencer et al., 1988) that "this therapeutic effect was restricted to female patients with schizophrenia or major affective disorders. The effect of family treatment on male patients with these diagnoses was minimal or slightly negative. In a group of patients with other diagnoses, the sex effect was reversed: male patients did better with the family treatment."

Russell et al. (1987) reported on the outcome of 80 patients (57 with anorexia nervosa and 23 with bulimia nervosa) who, upon discharge from a specialized unit (designed to restore their weight to normal), were assigned randomly to either family therapy or individual supportive therapy. One year later, follow-up studies revealed that family therapy was more effective than individual therapy with patients whose illness was not chronic and had not begun before the age of 19.

Chronic illnesses such as schizophrenia also benefit from family treatment. In one study, treatment was focused on the case-specific needs of the patients and their families by integrating individual and family psychotherapy and the use of therapeutic communities (Alanen et al., 1985). The authors conclude, "a family-centered approach is most successful when support was available to families and reinforced with individual psychotherapy."

Children

While not the primary scope of this chapter, the clinical principles underpinning managed care treatment of psychiatric and substance abuse disorders, apply even more cogently to the child and adolescent population. The literature for this age group has accumulated mainly in the public sector, where social and financial pressures have indeed been the mother of invention. Unfortunately, the very expensive private-sector treatment programs have generated precious little outcome research. Since the families covered under managed care are certainly no more disorganized or handicapped than those treated in the public sector, and as a rule less so, it would seem safe to assume that the favorable outcomes established for public sector recipients could be anticipated in the managed care environment.

The basic principles for children and adolescents are not different than for adults, except that even more attention must be focused on the social-surround and on normalizing the psychosocial environment of the identified patient. And more attention must be paid to the meaning of treatment setting and type upon the evolving self-identity of the child and adolescent, for this shapes and directs the entire future development of the individual. For an adult, being in a psychiatric hospital may be unpleasant, expensive, and of no benefit; for a child, it may confirm an emerging self-concept as a deviant, as someone that "even his own mother can't love"—or tolerate in her home.

There has been less attention in the literature to outpatient psychotherapy studies on children and adolescents (Casey and Berman, 1985) than on adults. Those that are available show no more than mildly positive effects. They all show that psychotherapy is least likely to be helpful to those with generalized conduct disorders, who account for the majority of the clientele in childhood and adolescence (Rutter and Giller, 1984).

The literature reports that neither behaviorally nor psychodynamically oriented inpatient and residential treatments for children and adolescents demonstrate superior outcomes to alternative programs. In addition, a number of articles substantiate iatrogenic, negative effects on self esteem, post-hospital adjustment, and family functioning (Rivlin and Wolfe, 1985; Winsbery et al., 1980). For day hospitals, there are generally positive effects, with fewer iatrogenic side effects, and with smoother reintegration into school and family (Kettlewell et al., 1985).

CONCLUSION

Mental health practitioners and academics can no longer ignore the clinical and social correctness of managed mental health approaches, for the economic power and the clinical imperatives that underlie managed mental health are compelling. Escalating costs have made change necessary; an enhanced diagnostic and treatment armamentarium and an adequate supply of trained professionals have made it possible. Our knowledge base, particularly in the biological area is richer than ever before.

And yet, mental health and substance abuse services continue to be viewed with skepticism by the general public and cynicism by the payors, all too aware of the waste and poor outcomes that plague it. This view will change when mental health practice, structure and resource allocation more closely match the state of our knowledge. Managed mental health represents an opportunity to bring this about.

REFERENCES

Alanen, Y.O., et al: Psychotherapeutically oriented treatment of schizophrenia: Results of 5-year follow-up. *Acta Psychiatrica Scandinavia, 71:*32–49, 1985.

Anderson, D.F.: Managed mental health care delivers the goods. Presented at the 1989 annual meeting of the American Psychiatric Association, San Francisco, California.

AuClaire, P., and Schwartz, I.M.: *An Evaluation of the Effectiveness of Intensive Home-Based Services as an Alternative to Placement for Adolescents and Their Families.* University of Minnesota, Hubert H. Humphrey Institute of Public Affairs, Center for Youth Policy, 1986.

Barer, M.L.: The low cost of universal access to healthcare in Canada. *Canadian Treasury Management Review,* August, 6–11, 1989.

Bengelsdorf, H., and Alden, D.C.: A mobile crisis unit in the psychiatric emergency room. *Hospital and Community Psychiatry, 38:*662–665, 1987.

Blackwell, B., Gutmann, M., and Gutmann, L.: Case review and quantity of outpatient care. *Am J Psychiatry, 145:*1003–1006, 1988.

Blouin, J., et al: Effects of patient characteristics and therapeutic techniques on crisis intervention outcome. *Psychiatric J of the University of Ottawa, 10:*153–157, 1983.

Borus, J.R., et al: The "offset effect" of mental health treatment on ambulatory medical care utilization and charges. Month-by-month and grouped-month analyses of a five-year study. *Arch Gen Psychiatry, 42:*573–80, 1985.

Borus, J.F., et al: Primary health care providers' recognition and diagnosis of mental disorders in their patients. *Gen Hosp Psychiatry, 10:*317–321, 1988.

Casey, R., and Berman, J.: The outcome of psychotherapy with children. *Psychological Bulletin, 98:*388–400, 1985.

Caton, C.L.M., and Gralnick, A.: A review of issues surrounding length of psychiatric hospitalization. *Hosp Comm Psychiatry, 38:*858–863, 1987.

Costello, E.J., et al: Psychopathology in pediatric primary care; the new hidden morbidity. *Pediatrics, 82:*415–424, 1988.

Costello, E.J., et al: Service utilization and psychiatric diagnosis in pediatric primary care: the role of the gatekeeper. *Pediatrics, 82:*435–441, 1988.

Diehr, P., Price K. and Martin, D.P.: Use of outpatient somatic health services by patients who use or need mental health services in three provider plans. *J Med Syst, 9:*389–400, 1985.

Drake, R.E., Gates, C., Whitaker, A., and Cotton, P.G.: Suicide among schizophrenics: a review. *Compr Psychiatry, 26:*90–100, 1985.

Epstein, L.H., et al: Long-term effects of family-based treatment of childhood obesity. *J of Consulting and Clinical Psychology, 55:*91–95, 1987.

Fisher, S.G.: Time-limited brief therapy with families: a one-year follow-up study. *Family Process, 23:*101–106, 1984.

Friedman, H., and Taub, H.A.: Extended follow-up study of the effects of brief psychological procedures in migraine therapy. *Am J of Clinical Hypnosis, 28:*27–33, 1985.

Galanter, M., Castaneda, R., and Ferman, J.: Substance abuse among general psychiatric patients: place of presentation, diagnosis, and treatment. *Am J of Drug and Alcohol Abuse, 14:*211–235, 1988.

Goldman, H.H., and Taube, C.A.: High users of outpatient mental health services, II: implications for practice and policy. *Am J Psychiatry, 145:*24–28, 1988.

Goldstein, J.M., et al: Identifying catastrophic psychiatric cases. *Med Care, 26:*790–798, 1988.

Hall, A., and Crisp, A.H.: Brief psychotherapy in the treatment of anorexia nervosa: Outcome at one year. *British J of Psychiatry, 151:*185–191, 1987.

Hass, G.L., et al: Inpatient family intervention: A randomized clinical trial: II Results at hospital discharge. *Archives of General Psychiatry, 45:*217–224, 1988.

Hayashida, et al: Comparative effectiveness and costs of inpatient and outpatient detoxification of patients with mild-to-moderate alcohol withdrawal syndrome. *N Eng J Med, 320:*358–364, 1989.

Heying, K.R.: Family-based in-home services for the severely emotionally disturbed child. *Child Welfare, 64:*519–527, 1985.

Hillman, A.L., Paul, M.V., and Kerstein, J.J.: How do financial incentives affect physicians' clinical decisions and the financial performance of health maintenance organizations? *N Eng J of Med, 321:*86–92, 1989.

Horowitz, M.J., et al: Comprehensive analysis of change after brief dynamic psychotherapy. *Am J Psychiatry, 143:*582–589, 1986.

Howard, K.L., et al: Patterns of psychotherapy utilization. *Am J. Psychiatry, 146:*775–778, 1989.

Husby, R., et al: Short-term dynamic psychotherapy: prognostic value of characteristics of patients studied by a 2-year follow-up of 39 neurotic patients. *Psychotherapy and Psychosomatics, 43:*8–16, 1985a.

Husby, R.: Short-term dynamic psychotherapy: a 5-year follow-up of 39 neurotic patients. *Psychotherapy and Psychosomatics, 43:*17–22, 1985b.

Julavits, W.F.: Psychiatric home care. An evolving legal standard. *Psychiatric Clinics of North America, 8:*577–586, 1985.

Kenney, K.C.: Research in mental health consultation: Emerging trends, issues, and problems. In Mannino, E.J., et al. (Eds): *Handbook of Mental Health Consultation,* Rockville, National Institute of Mental Health, 1986, pp 435–469.

Kettlewell, P.W., Jones, J.K., and Jones, R.H.: Adolescent partial hospitalization: Some preliminary outcome data. *Journal of Clinical Child Psychology, 14:*139–144, 1985.

Klerman, G.L.: Depressive disorders: Further evidence for increased medical morbidity and impairment of social functioning. *Arch Gen Psychiatry, 46:*856–858, 1989.

Klerman, G.L. and Weissman, M.M.: Increasing rates of depression. *JAMA, 361:* 2229–2234, 1989.

Langman-Dorwart, N. and Peebles, T.: A comprehensive approach to managed care for mental health. *Admin Ment Hlth, 15:*226–235, 1988.

Litman, G.K., and Topham, A.: Outcome studies on techniques in alcoholism treatment. *Recent Developments in Alcoholism, 1:*167–194, 1983.

Luft, H.S.: *Health Maintenance Organizations: Dimensions of Performance.* New York, John Wiley, 1981.

Luft, H.S.: HMO's and the quality of care. *Inquiry, 25:*147–156, 1988.

MacKenzie, K.R.: Recent developments in brief psychotherapy. *Hospital and Community Psychiatry, 39:*742–752, 1988.

Manning, W.G., Wells K.B., Benjamin, B.: Use of outpatient mental health services over time in a health maintenance organization and fee-for-service plans. *AM J Psychiatry, 144:*283–287, 1987.

McFarland, B.H., Freeborn, D.K., Mullooly, J.P., and Pope, C.R.: Utilization patterns among long-term enrollees in a prepaid group practice health maintenance organization. *Med Care, 23:*1221–1233, 1985.

McGuire, T.G. and Fairbank, A.: Patterns of mental health utilization over time in a fee-for-service population. *Am J Pub Hlth, 78:*134–136, 1988.

McKelvey, R.S.: A continuum of mental health care for children and adolescents. *Hospital and Community Psychiatry, 39:*870–873, 1988.

Melton, G.B.: Service models in child and adolescent mental health: what works for whom? Technical report to the Nebraska Department of Public Institutions, pursuant to Child and Adolescent Service System Program (CASSP) grant #MH39884-02 from the National Institute of Mental Health, 1986.

Mumford, E. et al: A new look at evidence about reduced cost of medical utilization following mental health treatment. *AM J Psychiatry, 141:*1145–1185, 1984.

Myers, J.K. et al.: Six-month prevalence of psychiatric disorders in three communities. *Arch Gen Psychiatry, 41:*959–967, 1984.

Nace, E.P.: Epidemiology of alcoholism and prospects for treatment. *Annual Review of Medicine, 35:*293–309, 1984.

Pang, J., Jr: Partial hospitalization: An alternative to inpatient care. *Psychiatric Clinics of North America, 8:*587–95, 1985.

Parker, S., and Knoll, J.L.: Partial Hospitalization: An update. *Am J Psychiatry, 147:*156–160, 1990.

Pelletier, L.R.: Psychiatric home care. *Journal of Psychosocial Nursing and Mental Health Services, 21:*22–27, 1988.

Piersma, H.L., and VanWingen, S.: A hospital-based crisis service for adolescents: a program description. *Adolescence, 23:*491–500, 1988.

Raphael, B.: Preventive intervention with the recently bereaved. *Archives of General Psychiatry, 34:*1450–462, 1983.

Reich, P.: Panic attacks and the risk of suicide. *N Eng J Med, 321:*1260–1261, 1989.

Rivlin, L.G., and Wolfe, M.: *Institutional Settings in Children's Lives.* New York, Wiley, 1985.

Robins, L.N., et al: Lifetime prevalence of specific psychiatric disorders in three sites. *Arch Gen Psychiatry, 41:*949–958, 1984.

Rosie, J.S.: Partial hospitalization: A review of recent literature. *Hosp and Community Psychiatry, 38:*1291–9, 1987.

Russell, G.F., et al: An evaluation of family therapy in anorexia nervosa and bulimia nervosa. *Archives of General Psychiatry, 44:*1047–1056, 1987.

Rutter, M., and Giller, H.: *Juvenile Delinquency: Trends and Perspectives.* New York, Guilford, 1984.

Santiago, J.M., McCall, P.F., and Bachrach, L.L.: Integrated services for chronic mental patients: theoretical perspective and experimental results. *General Hospital Psychiatry, 7:*309–315, 1985.

Saxe, L., et al: *Health Case Study 22: the Effectiveness and Costs of alcoholism Treatment.* Office of Technology Assessment, 1983.

Saxe, L. and Goodman, L.: *The Effectiveness of Outpatient vs. Inpatient Treatment: Updating the OTA Report.* Prepared for The Prudential Insurance Company, 1988.

Schene, A.H., and Gersons, V.P.: Effectiveness and application of partial hospitalization. *Acta Psychiatric Scan, 74:*335–340, 1986.

Schuckit, M.A., Schwel, M.G., and Gold, E.: Prediction of outcome in inpatient alcoholics. *J of Studies on Alcohol, 47:*151–155, 1986.

Services in Community Mental Health: Programs and Processes. Chapel Hill, University of North Carolina Press, 1985.

Shadle, M., and Christianson, J.B.: The organization of mental health care delivery in HMO's. *Admin Mental Hlth, 15:*201–225, 1988.

Shemo, J.P.: Cost-effectiveness of providing mental health services: The offset effect. *Int J Psychiatry Med, 15:*19–30, 1986.

Smith, M.L., Glass, G.C., and Miller, T.I.: *The Benefits of Psychotherapy.* Baltimore, Johns Hopkins University Press, 1980.

Soreff, S.M.: Indications for home treatment. *Psychiatric Clinics of North America, 8:*563–575, 1985.

Spencer, J.H., Jr., et al: A randomized clinical trial of inpatient family intervention: Effects at 6 months and 18 months follow-ups. *AM J Psychiatry, 145:*1115–1121, 1988.

Stein, R.E., and Jessop, D.J.: Does pediatric home care make a difference for children with chronic illness? Findings from the Pediatric Ambulatory Care Treatment Study. *Pediatrics, 73:*845–853, 1984.

Subramanian, K.: Reducing child abuse through respite center intervention. *Child Welfare, 64:*501–509, 1985.

Svedlund, J., and Sjodin, I.: A psychosomatic approach to treatment in the irritable bowel syndrome and peptic ulcer disease with aspects of the design of clinical trials. *Scandinavian Journal of Gastroenterology, Supplement 109:*147–151, 1985.

Taube, C.A., et al: High users of outpatient mental health services: definition and characteristics. *Am J Psychiatry 145:*19–24, 1988.

Tessler, R.C.: Continuity of care and client outcome. *Psychosocial Rehabilitation Journal, 11:*39–53, 1987.

Viney, L.L., et al: Sex differences in the psychological reactions of medical and surgical patients to crisis intervention counseling: Sauce for the goose may not be sauce for the gander. *Social Science and Medicine, 20:*1199–1205, 1985.

Weissman, M.M., et al: Suicidal ideation and suicide attempts in panic disorder and attacks. *N Eng J Med, 321:*1209–1214, 1989.

Wells, K.B., et al: The functioning and well-being of depressed patients: Results from the medical outcomes study. *JAMA, 262:*914–919, 1989.

Wells, K.B., et al: Detection of depressive disorder for patients receiving prepaid or fee-for-service care: Results from the medical outcomes study. *JAMA, 23:*3298–3302, 1989.

Wells, K.B., Manning, W.G., and Benjamin, B.: Use of outpatient mental health services in HMO and fee-for-service plans: results from a randomized controlled trial. *Health Serv Res, 21:*453–74, 1986.

Willard, J.R., et al: Suicide in a psychiatric emergency room population. *Am J Psychiatry, 140:*459–462, 1983.

Winsbery, B.G., et al: Home versus hospital care of children with behavior disorders: A controlled investigation. *Archives of General Psychiatry, 37:*413–418, 1980.

Chapter 12

ETHICAL ISSUES IN MANAGED MENTAL HEALTH

Stephen R. Blum

The increasing presence of managed care in the American market-place is, historically, an extension of social policies that seek to increase the effectiveness of health care services (Bayer, Feldman and Reich, 1981). The managed care era is one that will almost certainly contain important ethical issues for virtually all those involved in the process: policy planners, corporate providers of mental health benefits, managed care firms, clinicians, and, not least of all, consumers. Because there is increasing concern that mental health services are neither as effective, efficient or as equitable as they could be, managed mental health programs are developing rapidly. They are likely to provide fertile ground for the examination of the value assumptions and applied ethical decisions that inform managed mental health services.

In their briefest form, the ethical issues that arise with the development of managed mental health services have to do with the nature of the relationship between the money spent on such services and the quality of care provided. The arguments by those who oppose the growth of managed mental health care are similar to the ones made by the opponents of Independent Practice Associations, Health Maintenance Organizations, Preferred Provider Organizations and their progeny (Boaz, 1988). In essence, they state that the quality of patient care will or must decrease as oversight and controls on expenditures increase, and as the money spent on care decreases: thus, to manage care is to threaten its quality. The opposite side claims that the quality of care in managed settings is not inferior, but is at least equal to, or better than, unmanaged care such as in fee-for-service.

This argument has raged for as long as there have been alternatives to fee-for-service arrangements. Given the vagaries associated with defining "quality of care," it is likely to continue, perhaps for some time. The issue here is the tension between those whose ideology and financial incentives are to do more, and those who are motivated to do less. The translation of these contrary positions into mental health services has consequences that raise ethical issues. Given this tension, what are the characteristics of patient care in managed mental health settings, and what are their ethical dimensions?

This chapter first examines some contextual issues, including the utility of applied health care ethics using a multi-perspective framework; allocative decisions as a basic and ongoing part of the distribution of American health care resources; and the business of managing new behaviors for health providers and consumers. Second, the chapter discusses some ethical issues that arise when mental health services are provided under any one of a number of arrangements collectively called "managed care." These issues include possible compromises to patient autonomy; possible compromises to the professional autonomy of mental health providers; difficulties associated with informed consent and confidentiality that can arise in managed mental health arrangements; and, threats to confidentiality that may arise because of the "double agent" problem.

Managed Mental Health and Applied Health Care Ethics

For purposes of this chapter, applied health care ethics is the discipline that critically examines the value assumptions and conflicts that are present, even if unacknowledged or unexamined, in the managed mental health enterprise. Virtually all social policy planning takes place within a dynamic and often ambiguous socio-political environment. To acknowledge this is to assume that the development and implementation of new social policies, such as managed care, are *always* contextuated with assumptions that represent values and beliefs about what is right or just or fair. There is an inextricable ethical component in all social policy although the ethical dimension may be unrecognized or unacknowledged (Brown, 1990; Callahan, 1987; Veatch and Branson, 1976).

Applied health care ethics seeks to critically assess the value choices that are an integral part of policy and program development. Such choices are often indebted to and rely on various ethical theories, albeit often only implicitly. The goal of applied health care ethics is to render explicit and critically examine the value issues and choices that arise in actual service delivery settings to actual persons seeking or receiving services. Applied health care ethics examines human choices that have non-trivial consequences, not only for policy planners, entrepreneurs, and program developers, but also, importantly, for those who provide and consume services (Calabresi and Bobbitt, 1978; Daniels, 1988).

The assessment of human conduct is the realm of applied ethics; such assessment seeks to analyze and respond to the question "What is right conduct or action?" The design of health services, such as managed care, that allocate and thus designate limits of service should be subject to ethical reflection and assessment. In this way, applied health care ethics may lead to the development of suggested standards of conduct for those involved.

Managed care, briefly put, places new constraints on access to health services. These new constraints seek to: (1) reduce or eliminate unnecessary services, and thus, (2) reduce the costs of care, while, at the same time, (3) maintaining or increasing its effectiveness. These three inter-related goals have been central to the rhetoric and the aspirations of the health planning movement in America for the past two or more decades. They are the major outcomes sought by many federal and state health policy initiatives that have sought to encourage capitated service delivery in HMOs, and to contain costs through such efforts as the certificate of need process and DRGs.

Managed care should be seen as a further step to refine "utilization management" strategies. Initially, these efforts were primarily directed to inpatient hospital care. The Institute of Medicine's 1989 *Report of the Committee on Utilization Management by Third Parties*

> ... adopted a relatively narrow definition of utilization management as "a set of techniques used by or on behalf of purchasers of health benefits to manage health care costs by influencing patient care decision-making through case-by-case assessments of the appropriateness of care prior to its provision. . . . The major forms of utilization management are (1) prior review of proposed medical services through such means as preadmission or admission review for elective or emergency hospital admissions, continued stay review for hospitalized patients, and pre-procedure review for selected inpatient and outpatient services; and (2) high-cost case management. Recently the focus has begun to include case-by-case assessments of the medical need for particular procedures (Field and Gray, 1989).

In the context of mental health services, the term managed care is used here to describe those arrangements, offered almost exclusively by private firms, to providers of health benefits in order to influence patient care decision-making and achieve the three goals mentioned above:

more appropriate utilization of services; more control of costs, and the maintenance (or, in the ideal, the improvement) of quality.

In contrast to a number of other "developed" nations, in America there is no legal right to health services. The American health and mental health system is one where eligibility for services has been dependent in good measure on the ability to pay (Starr, 1982). With the not insignificant exception of voluntary or government programs, health care in America is best understood as a large, powerful, and growing set of private business enterprises (Estes, 1982; Relman, 1980; Veatch and Branson, 1976). Thus, to speak of managed mental health is, largely, to speak of mental health business enterprises (Kongstvedt, 1989), and profit as an important goal of such (Institute of Medicine, 1986).

For-profit health and mental health care are not *automatically* ethically suspect. There is some evidence to suggest that the differences between for-profit and non-profit care providers may not be as significant as might be supposed (Brock and Buchanan, 1986). The ethical issues that arise in managed mental health may occur in either proprietary or non-profit settings, and their prevalence in one setting or another is a matter of ongoing debate (Relman and Reinhardt, 1986). There may well be circumstances in the business environment which could exacerbate ethical issues as they arise in managed mental health care (Fein, 1990). A detailed examination of that issue—along with the related questions of the need for standards of corporate behavior initiated either voluntarily by managed care firms or under the aegis of legislative and regulatory activity—awaits a more thorough knowledge of the operating environment of this relatively new and rapidly growing segment of the health care industry (Institute of Medicine, 1989; Field and Gray, 1989; Staver, 1989).

The rapid evolution of managed mental health and medical care in general brings with it a set of givens. They are the starting point for an understanding of managed care and include the fact that:

1. Managed mental health strategies are not designed to address major ethical and health policy concerns such as the already existent limitations in the mental health services delivery system. Managed mental health does not address, for example, issues of equity and access to mental health services for all socio economic groups nor the maldistribution of service providers. Managed mental health tacitly accepts the very real limits of the existing delivery system. It

does not seek any significant reconfiguration of the system that
would, for example, provide mental health services for those that
are in need but who are not now served adequately (e.g., many of
the poor, many of the elderly, many who have, or will have, AIDS,
etc.). Managed care tends to work with the system as it is, not with
how it might or should be.

2. For managed mental health the issue is not who receives care — that
   decision has already been made by the benefit provider (e.g., the
   employer) before contracting with the managed care firm. For
   managed care the issue is what kind, by whom and how much care
   is provided. Managed care generally involves superimposing new
   forms of oversight and services onto an already-existing population
   of eligibles. It attempts to provide care that is equal or better in
   quality than the patient has received in the past, for less money.
   The focus is on the intensity of care, and the setting in which it is
   provided. It is not generally within the purview of managed care to
   expand (or contract) the pool of eligibles who might receive care.
   Managed care is thus an addition to an already-existing array of
   services.

It can be argued that ethical considerations are of importance in
managed mental health because they are often unexamined and because
they arise in a number of settings, some of them institutional and some
in practitioners' offices. In all of these settings, and perhaps especially in
institutional settings, the phenomenon of what Kenneth Arrow called
"informational inequality" is pervasive (Arrow, 1963). By this term,
Arrow meant that the person who has become, or seeks to become, a
patient is usually deeply (and sometimes abjectly) dependent upon the
provider. Often the choice of treatment is provider-driven, and there is a
relative lack of consumer "freedom of choice" with regard to what services patients receive — the choices are made for them. These choices are
made either by a provider acting alone, or, in managed care arrangements,
by a provider acting in concert with a care manager or managed care
firm. Informational inequality is a structural feature of virtually all
health care services, and perhaps even more so in mental health. It has
significant consequences for the relationship between clinician and
consumer. One concomitant of this inequality is paucity of information-
sharing that takes place between consumer and provider.

In medicine, and in mental health services, this structural inequality often leads to a form of non-communication that has been characterized as the "the silent world of doctor and patient" (Katz, 1984). In such a world, rational choice-making by the consumer is rare, and consumer fear is prevalent. Vladeck (1981) notes the consequences of this state of events:

> Consumers have sought the kind of health insurance that they have, not because they wish to act irrationally in the aggregate economic sense, but precisely because they don't wish to be forced to make rational trade-offs when they are confronted with medical care consumption decisions. No matter how we draw our curves or shape our abstract arguments, the elemental fact is that medical care is about living and dying, something considered by many to be of a rather different character than the purchase of tomatoes. The primary characteristic of most consumers of medical care most of the time is that they are scared. They are scared of dying, or disfigurement, or permanent disability, and these are serious matters. It is hardly fair to expect any of us to make rational decisions about matters of such import.

In managed care arrangements, the "silent world" may not only be between clinician and consumer: increasingly, there is another key player, the "manager" of care. What was heretofore an often "silent" and thus ethically troubling dyad has become, with the addition of the manager of care, a potentially even more ethically troublesome triad. Informational inequality tends to grow more acute when the client or patient is particularly vulnerable, as is often the case with persons seeking mental health services. Their ailment, because it is often not "physical," and therefore less visible, may be more fearsome and more mysterious. Managed mental health services have the potential to either help decrease informational inequality and lessen the vulnerability experienced by patients, or, of course, such arrangements also have the potential to make these circumstances even more difficult than they were in an "unmanaged care" environment.

Feelings of vulnerability, however, may not lie wholly in the province of the patient or consumer but extend to providers as well when their autonomy with regard to clinical decisions is limited, without the exchange of adequate information. Vulnerable providers may be individual clinicians who are affiliated with or in the employ of a managed care firm (Berenson, 1989; Buie, 1989; Staver, 1989). They may also be the administrators and employees of inpatient facilities that operated in the past without managed care oversight (Larkin, 1989).

Indeed, the majority of the membership of an entire profession may feel frustrated by and vulnerable to organizational changes such as those that come with managed care. This is apparently the case with medicine now (Belkin, 1990), and it may well be happening with mental health professionals (Berenson, 1989). Some of the scenarios for the future of managed mental health are not likely to ease their concerns. According to Brag (1989):

> ... the prepaid sector of health care delivery is in the midst of a period of rapid growth, a period that is likely to continue until this mode of health care emerges as the dominant one in this country. An equally dramatic transformation is likely to occur in the manner in which mental health care is delivered; forces already in motion point to the day when short-term therapy, frequently in group form, will supplant long-term, one-on-one therapy, which has been the tradition of the past. Eventually the concept of peer self-help, already in place in such groups as Alcoholics Anonymous, may actually set aside the need for professional mental health practitioners.

Managed mental health arrangements are designed to alter some of the ways in which patients and providers interact. Changes in the relationship between provider and consumer are at the core of what managed mental health is, and what it seeks to accomplish. Under managed care, the mental health services dyad has become a triad. That triad will behave differently, for it has different assumptions, goals and values, than did the "unmanaged" client-provider dyad (Altman and Rosenthanl, 1989).

The ethical issues assessed here form part of what Brody calls a "moral pluralistic casuistry" (Brody, 1988). Such a framework explicitly presumes values and beliefs about "right action" to often be in conflict. Further, such a framework presumes the inappropriateness of ethical monism: there is no *single* coherent set of moral and philosophical assumptions that, like a template, apply to any health care quandary. No one purview alone can provide reliable and useful recommendations for appropriate understanding and "right action." Multiple perspectives are a prerequisite for a better understanding of what actions we ought to take.

The issues described above—applied health care ethics using a multi-perspective framework, concern for allocative decisions, and the business of creating new behaviors for providers and consumers— form the context for an examination of four central ethical issues that arise within managed mental health. Foremost among these is respect for patient autonomy and how it is potentially redefined under managed care.

Respect for Patient Autonomy

Respect for patient autonomy means that health care decisions must respect human worth and enhance self-determination. The principle of respect for autonomy holds that self-worth has, as a prerequisite, respect for self-determined actions or choices (Beauchamp and Childress, 1989; Veatch, 1981). Autonomous choices however, can be subordinated, waived, or over-ridden (Childress, 1990):

> It is important for the moral life that people be competent, be informed and act voluntarily. But they may choose, for example, to yield their first-order decisions (that is, decisions about the rightness or wrongness about a particular mode of conduct). For example they may yield to their physicians when medical treatment is proposed. . . . Abdication of first-order autonomy appears to involve heteronomy, that is, rule by others. However, if a person autonomously chooses to yield first-order decision making to a professional . . . that person has exercised what may be called second-order autonomy. People who are subservient to a professional . . . may lack first-order autonomy . . . because they have exercised and continue to exercise second-order autonomy in selecting the professional or institution to which they choose to be subordinate. Hence, in those cases, respect for second-order autonomy is central, even though their first-order choices are heteronomous.

Threats to self-determination take place in settings where autonomy is diminished, as is almost always the case within health care. Childress (1990) also suggests that

> The principle of respect for autonomy can be stated negatively as "it is [prima facie] wrong to subject the actions (including choices) of others to controlling influence." This principle provides the justificatory basis for the right to make autonomous decisions. . . . This negative formulation focuses on avoidance of controlling influences, including coercion and lying. However, the principle of respect for autonomy also has clear positive implications in the context of certain relationships, including health care relationships.

The treatment process begins with a person who is often vulnerable, suffering from dis-ease, as well as from some degree of informational inequality. Respect for personal autonomy may be compromised during the transformational process that occurs when a person becomes a "patient," a "case," a DSM–III description, or a "client" (Brody, 1988; Katz, 1982; Kleinman, 1988). If the process of becoming a patient, in and of itself, threatens self-determination, what might be the additional effect of becoming a patient whose care is under the purview of a "manager" or a managed care program? As real as the threats to personal autonomy are in the traditional dyadic arrangement, they are potentially exacerbated by the entry of a third party whose mission is to add an oversight role to the traditional provider-patient dyad. Third party payors have been a fact of life in American health care for as long as there have been health insurance programs. But the emergence of managed care as well as the virtual demise of unquestioned fee-for-service retrospective billing arrangements, the evolution of capitation arrangements and the entry of the private sector into the business of managed care have all combined to change the historic dyad into a complex triad. The addition of third parties to managing and paying for treatment means that people other than the patient and the clinician have a voice, perhaps a controlling one, in the treatment process.

Often at risk in the traditional dyad, patient autonomy may be the recipient of beneficial oversight under managed care. Patients will almost certainly benefit, for example, from participation in a care management arrangement that seeks to ensure that their mental health care benefits are appropriately and judiciously used. This might well be the case, to use a common managed care example, where an alcohol-dependent patient is provided quality care on an outpatient basis rather than in a costly and often unnecessary 28-day inpatient program that uses up benefits inappropriately.

There are risks to the personal autonomy of patients in managed care settings. Managed care adds personnel to the treatment arena whose ultimate task is not to actually provide care, but to oversee that care in ways that meet multiple agendas. These agendas include quality assurance, utilization review, and, where appropriate, providing less intensive forms of treatment in order to gain economic advantage for the payor and profit for the managed care firm. The insertion of these third-party interests *may* serve as a bureaucratic and paternalistic impediment to the personal autonomy of the patient. It is difficult enough to cope with the ethical implications of clinician paternalism; the special interests of third-party payors and managers may well exacerbate the dangers and difficulties. This could compromise the fragile enterprise of autonomy-maintenance, one that should be central to *any* organizational configuration for the provision of mental health services (Brown, 1990).

In light of these potential difficulties, safeguards should be developed to guard against threats to patient autonomy that may occur under managed care. At a minimum, they should include the creation of systems, by the managed mental health provider, the employer and employees to be certain that decisions about care include provisions for due process, exceptions and appeals. These should be built into the managed care program from its inception, subject to review and modification on a regular basis. Managed care providers, like the administrators of all complex social service systems, must assume that their procedures and decisions will always be subject to error. Ways must exist inside the structure of managed mental health care to recognize such fallibility, and to have a process for quickly and compassionately rectifying mistakes. Systems that do not allow for such a process will verify procedures that are ethically inappropriate.

Threats to the Autonomy of Providers

While the principle of respect for autonomy in applied health care ethics has almost always been focused on the individual patient (e.g., Beauchamp and Childress, 1989; Childress, 1990), the development of managed care strategies has brought with it a concern about the autonomy of the health care provider as well. What are the ethical dimensions of this concern?

There is little question that the role of health care provider has changed rapidly in the past decade. As part of an effort to assess and improve effectiveness and, at the same time, to control costs, health care managers have implemented a number of strategies designed to monitor and assess that which was, in the past, largely free from such efforts. These have included programs to attempt to comparatively assess the adequacy and costs of care. In managed mental health this takes many forms, ranging from preadmission reviews, to continuing treatment authorizations, concurrent review and the use of "screens" (increasingly computerized), designed to determine the appropriateness of a treatment plan. Each of these can be said to stand between the clinician/ patient relationship. It was the traditional relationship, however, that was a causal part of the failings many believe to be central to the traditional mental health system. That system did little or nothing to address a panoply of important mental health policy issues including the maldistribution of services, provider-driven utilization and cost increases and questionable quality/cost effectiveness.

As the costs of mental health care have continued to rise, third party payors have come to question the continuing growth of mental health expenditures and the outcomes of care. The particular questions most often posed by managed care have to do with the locus, intensity and duration of treatment. With regard to locus of care, the question is whether relatively expensive inpatient care is most effective for particular conditions and justifies the cost. With regard to the duration of treatment, the major question is whether shorter lengths of stay and treatment regimens result in equal or better treatment outcomes than longer ones.

There are very real social and economic consequences of the continuing cost spiral of mental health services. But there are also consequences for those mental health professionals who see themselves as "caught in the middle" between a patient-centered ethic that seeks the best care for the individual patient and their perception of increasing "interference" from third parties who demand explanation, justification and oversight in order to authorize payment for services.

The rapid growth of third-party payors and managed care, with their stratagems for increased provider accountability, has resulted in series of significant changes in the practice patterns of physicians (Friedson, 1970). We may well be in the midst of a change in how medicine and the other health service professionals are defined. These changes have been the subject of analysis by a number of observers (McKinley and Stoeckle, 1988). Three of the most important are:

1. **Autonomy over the terms and content of work** that had been largely controlled by the individual practitioner is now controlled more so by owners or administrators with their own organizational constraints and motivations, including the earning of profit. More than one half of American physicians are now employees. The number who are self-employed continues to decline as younger physicians enter practice in corporate or other settings where they are employees (Altman and Rosenthanl, 1990).

2. **The clinical and fiduciary relationship with patients.** Patient "ownership" had, in the past, been largely under the control of the solo practi-

tioner. Now, more and more patients are members of organizations that have managed health and mental health benefits. These organizations and managers largely determine the standards for what will be treated, how, by whom, and the extent to which treatment will be reimbursed.

3. **Remuneration.** In the past the number of hours worked, how much was earned and the utilization of ancillary services (e.g., consultation, laboratory, etc.) were largely determined by the individual practitioner. This is less and less the case under managed care arrangements where provider remuneration is determined or at least significantly influenced by a third party. Remuneration also comes much more frequently in the form of a salary from an employer (McKinley and Arches, 1985).

Ethical concerns about provider autonomy have a different foundation than do those affecting patient decision-making and self-determination. Yet, as the fears and claims of increased infringement upon provider autonomy grow, there may be some parallels between the two. In both, for example, the claim is made that interference with autonomy results in treating a person as a means rather than an end; that threats to the autonomy of practitioner and patient both result in increased paternalistic intervention into the treatment process, no matter how beneficent such intervention may be. Increasingly, providers argue that such interventions can delay, impede, or change a treatment plan, with a negative effect on the quality of care. Some of these professionals claim that patient care in such arrangements suffers through the intervention of third parties. This view holds that the autonomous clinical judgment of the provider is threatened, to one degree or another, under any form of managed care. The threats, so this view holds, are both to the quality of care for patients and to the quality of the professional lives of mental health providers.

In all of these claims by providers little is said about the decline of professional prerogatives, not the least of which may be income, that often accompanies the involvement of third parties in the treatment relationship. Some observers suggest that it is this decline of prerogatives and the consequent loss of power and/or income that is really the major issue. In an interview with the *New York Times,* health economist Uwe Reinhardt stated why he thinks there will be a continuing impetus to arrangements such as managed care: "Physicians have lived like kids in a candy store. We, the payors, want the key back" (Altman and

Rosenthanl, 1990). Others as well appear to have little sympathy for the complaints of practitioners that their autonomy has been imperiled. They believe that "getting the key back" means a level of accountability heretofore unseen in American health care. Given the issues of cost, access, and quality, it is a level of accountability that many payors, believe is long overdue.

If managed mental health's efforts are to be judged successful, it will be because they have maintained or reduced service costs while maintaining or improving quality. The single most effective way to do so is to provide care that accomplishes treatment goals in less time and in less expensive settings. Such treatment reduces inpatient utilization by avoiding admissions and reducing lengths of stay when inpatient care is appropriate. In outpatient care, it means a greater emphasis on short-term psychotherapy.

Accomplishment of these objectives could very well result in a loss of income for the (non-salaried) mental health provider. Absent an increase in utilization from "unmanaged" clients, or other marketing, pricing or diversification strategies, this loss of income may be translated as a threat to the professional autonomy of clinicians and/or inpatient facilities. Insofar as the control of costs through managed care do not impair quality, then such undertakings are not unethical, the claims of loss of professional autonomy notwithstanding. What would raise ethical questions, however, would be rhetoric from providers about "imperiled" quality of care when what is actually declining or imperiled is their control or profit. From the perspective of applied health care ethics, health care is too frequently characterized by a patina of language ostensibly patient-loyal and patient-centered. Often, however, there are other issues at stake: professional power, prestige, and income. These are all very human propensities, but their exercise is rarely in the best interest of patients.

Organizational self-interest, greed and poor management are all possible outcomes of the rapid growth of managed mental health. Each would have significant negative consequences for patient care, and to the extent that they were willfully undertaken, they would be clearly unethical. The risks are real—the history of "the new medical industrial complex" and its progeny should make us vigilant about them (Bayer, Feldman and Reich, 1981; Relman, 1981; Starr, 1980). But while real, these risks are not necessary—they are not part and parcel of the conceptual underpinnings and the value assumptions that make up the managed care enterprise.

In mental health services, the absence of strong criteria for diagnosing and treating a number of mental disorders and for the amount of treatment needed is widely acknowledged. This is at least part of the reason that mental health is not included in the DRG cost-containment program. The ethical high-road for managed mental health as an enterprise will be taken if clinician judgments are respected such that when the managed care firm has questions about the treatment plan that could result in overriding such judgments, such a decision would only be made after careful consultation with the clinician. The central decision criterion should be based on what is in the best interest of the patient. Ethical professional practice, inside or outside the managed mental health arena, demands no less (Dougherty, 1989; Dyer, 1988).

Informed Consent

The ethical considerations of informed consent in health care, like those of respect for autonomy, are considered to be person-centered: patients have the right to be informed about their health so that their ability to exercise their own judgment is enhanced. This ethical precept is a central feature of the applied health care ethics literature.

> Virtually all medical and research codes of ethics hold that physicians and research investigators must obtain informed consent of patients and subjects before undertaking procedures. These consent measures have been designed to enable autonomous choices by patients and subjects, but they serve other functions as well, including the protection of patients and subjects against harm and the encouragement of medical professionals to act responsibly in their interactions with patients and subjects (Beauchamp and Childress, 1989).

Informed consent is not a product or thing (e.g., a signed "consent slip"), it is a process. The goal of such a process is to adequately provide information to patients (or in some carefully delineated circumstances to a duly appointed proxy) in order that they may anticipate whether they wish to consent to treatment (Wojcik, 1978). The elements that are necessary, but not always sufficient for informed consent include:

> (1) a fair explanation of the procedures or treatments, (2) a description of discomforts and risks, (3) a description of expected benefits, (4) disclosure of alternative procedures, (5) an offer to answer any inquiries, (6) an instruction that the person is free to withdraw consent

and discontinue participation in the project or activity, and (7) a
statement that withdrawal will not result in loss of benefits or prejudice
treatment. These are but minimal standards. It cannot be presumed
that once these requirements are met the physician or investigator has
no further obligations to the patient or experimental subject (Dyer,
1988).

Just how the informed consent process should be undertaken with
competent patients seeking mental health services has been a subject of
controversy for some time (Keith-Spiegel and Koocher, 1985; Monahan,
1980; Dyer, 1988). There are those clinicians, for example, who claim that
the need for an absolute arena of trust in the psychotherapeutic process
is, or could be, vitiated by any such conversations that would provide the
patient with the elements of informed consent. These mental health
providers claim that their work is substantially different from the practice of medicine, and that the criteria for informed consent should be
relaxed or abandoned as untenable, and undesirable as well, in mental
health settings.

Alternatively, a strong claim can be made that the process of informed
consent for treatment is at least as important in mental health as it is in
medicine. In its own way, mental health treatment can be as deeply
"invasive" as medical care, if less obviously so. Some would argue that
the need for informed consent in mental health is paramount, given the
need to preserve autonomous choices and the vulnerability that many
patients experience.

The informed consent issues, as well as the related ones of confidentiality
are more complex in a managed care environment. Managed care arrangements often include pre-authorizations for treatment. In such circumstances, information about a prospective patient may be shared on the
basis of implied or *deemed* consent before treatment has begun. Clinical
information about the presenting complaint, and perhaps a preliminary
estimate of its severity must be shared with the care managers in order
to secure authorization to begin treatment. Are prospective patients
informed and have they always given their consent for the release of such
information? Does pre-treatment authorization somehow redefine the
traditional understanding of informed consent, and, if it does, what
are the consequences for patient autonomy, for the maintenance of
confidentiality, and for the treatment process itself? In health care ethics,
the concept of *implied* consent is typically applied only in emergency
situations. Are we to assume that pre-authorization procedures man-

dated by managed care require the implied consent of the person seeking treatment? If this is the case, why be concerned about it?

Managed care inserts a new player, the care manager, into the consent
and confidentiality process. Generally, the manager approves or disap-
proves care based on information that does not come directly from the
patient and may or may not be confidential in the eyes of the person
seeking treatment. The person seeking to be a patient is not directly
included in the pre-authorization process, and is not part of conversations about symptoms, needs and treatment alternatives. Is the pre-
authorization process, for example, actually based upon deemed or
implied consent, or is that the assumption that the manager and the
clinician, acting together, have made?

What appears to be the case in these circumstances is that the third
party payor and/or manager have the power to decide on treatment but
may not have direct knowledge of the prospective patient's wishes. It
may also be that the person seeking help is only dimly aware of the locus
of the decision, who is making it and on what basis. To help with these
problems, the payors, clinicians, managers of care and consumers of
managed mental health services should have answers to at least the
following questions:

1. Where are the records kept of the pre-treatment authorization and
   managed care process, and what do they contain?
2. Who has access to such information?
3. How are potential patients informed about the pre-authorization
   process, and the role of the managed care firm?
4. How can the managed care firm directly include the potential
   patient in the pre-authorization "loop"? Can people who have been
   the subject of discussion with a managed care firm access their
   records from the firm?
5. How can the employer/payor, the clinician, and the managed care
   firm act in concert to create an informed consent process that
   protects patient autonomy and confidentiality?

It should not be the norm to have these questions answered and
decisions made out of sight of consumers "for their own good" by third
parties. To every extent possible, discussions and decisions about them
should be made with the person most directly affected: the consumer.

The "Double Agent" Problem

Applied health care ethics has long considered the so-called "double agent" problem whereby clinicians seek to be singularly loyal to the patient but, at the same time, are in the employ of an organization that has its own needs and expectations (Bloch and Chodoff, 1981; Chodoff, 1981; Keith-Spiegel and Koocher, 1985; Levine, 1972).

Managed mental health care is the contemporary version of the double agent problem, writ large. Questions about professional behavior under circumstances of "divided loyalties" are integral to employee assistance and other occupational mental health programs; they confront any mental health program where the payor (usually, the employer) wants patient/ employee information. This wish for information is understandable, but it is ethically indefensible and if provided, would doom the entire effort. Managed mental health care efforts to maintain confidentiality (and thus autonomy) are threatened by those payor-employers who believe that they have a need, and possibly a "right," to information about the treatment of their employees, at least insofar as it relates to job performance.

Here, as elsewhere, the tradition of strict confidentiality in the mental health arena must remain constant; to do otherwise places the therapeutic activity in serious jeopardy and negates the very premises of the program itself. Such a program could not and should not be trusted as a place to seek treatment by employees. There are, of course, limited exceptions to a policy of strict confidentiality; they are already part of the law or central to the ethics of the treatment itself (for example, a clinician's perception of a real threat to do violence to a fellow employee).

But the double agent problem does not end with questions of confidentiality, serious as they may be. The matter grows more complex in the managed mental health environment with regard to determining who the "client" is and also who the "agent" is. The actors include (1) the patient, (2) the clinician, (3) the employer/payor, and (4) the mental health manager. The scenario is as follows:

1. **The patient** seeks confidential and effective treatment, and may well prefer that all aspects of that treatment be a matter for discussion only with the clinician. Given the prevalence of third-party payment arrangements, patients should be told as part of the informed consent process, as proximate to the start of therapy as possible, that there is information that the clinician must tell others in order to assure coverage

of the care provided. The patient should be told what that information consists of, to whom it will be given and should give explicit consent for it to be communicated.

2. **The clinician** seeks to keep the needs and wishes of the patient uppermost and yet to behave in a manner deemed appropriate by the care manager and payor. The clinician must advocate on behalf of the patient, knowing that it is clinical judgment that must be key in decisions about treatment. This advocacy role may be threatened by the clinician's referral base and income.

3. **The employer/payor** has a fiduciary relationship with the patient (as an employee who receives benefits), the clinician, albeit perhaps indirectly through the care manager and the managed care firm. The expectations of the employer/payor include obtaining quality care for the patient at an appropriate cost. Yet, this request for cost-effective care may be regarded by the clinician as a "threat to professional autonomy." From the perspective of the employer/payor and the care manager there is a need to increase clinician accountability and thus control the costs of what had hitherto been both largely unaccountable and increasingly expensive.

4. **The care manager** seeks to please the employer/payor by helping to provide quality care, containing costs and, at the same time, maintaining a satisfactory relationship with clinicians. The manager seeks to be sensitive to the needs of each of the other three parties, but, ultimately, would not be in business were it not for the contracts given them by employers/payors. If the wishes of the employer/payor for high quality and cost containment are not congruent, the manager of care is out of business.

In order to maintain accountability and to control costs, managers of care are likely to be seen at least by some clinicians as intrusive. That perception will often be correct. From an ethical perspective, the question is how managed mental health can give primacy to patients in a manner that allows all parties to the process not to be disabled by the reality of double agent processes and problems. An ongoing ethical assessment of this issue and others related to complicating loyalties is both the responsibility and the challenge of all those who are double agents in the growing world of managed mental health. This is particularly important for those who set the limits on care, for the employer/payor and the care manager.

Conclusion

The advent and evolution of managed mental health has brought with it a host of ethical issues, some of which have been explored here. It could be argued that these issues are not new, that they are not caused by managed mental health, but rather that managed mental health simply highlights and exacerbates them. It is true that many of the issues are central to applied health care ethics under virtually any configuration for mental health services, managed or otherwise. Specific to managed mental health or not, the ethical issues are real and important to everyone involved in mental health services. The success of managed mental health must be judged not only on the basis of its quality and cost effectiveness but on the extent to which these ethical issues are addressed and resolved satisfactorily. To do otherwise would endanger an enterprise from which all sectors of society can benefit.

REFERENCES

Altman, L.A., and Rosenthanl, E: Changes in medicine bring pain to healing profession. *New York Times, 139:*20–21, 1990.

Arrow, K.J.: Uncertainty and the welfare economics of medical care. *American Economic Review,* 53:941–973, 1963, cited in Relman, Arnold S.: The new medical-industrial complex. *New England Journal of Medicine, 303:*963–970, 1980.

Bayer, R., Feldman, S., and Reich, W.: *Ethical Issues in Mental Health Policy and Administration.* Washington, DC, U.S. Department of Health and Human Services, National Institute of Mental Health, DHHS Publication No. ADM-81-1116, 1981.

Beauchamp, T.L. and Childress, J.F.: *Principles of Biomedical Ethics,* 3rd ed. New York, Oxford, 1989.

Belkin, L.: Many in medicine see rules sapping profession's morale. *New York Times, 139:*A-1, A-9, 1990.

Berenson, R.A.: A physician's reflections. *Hastings Center Report, 19:*12–18, 1989.

Bloch, S. and Chodoff, P. (Eds.): *Psychiatric Ethics.* New York, Oxford, 1981.

Boaz, J.T.: *Delivering Mental Healthcare: A Guide for HMOs.* Chicago, Pluribus, 1988.

Brock, D.W. and Buchanan, A.: Ethical issues in for-profit health care. In Gray, B. H. (Ed.): *For-Profit Enterprise in Health Care.* Washington, DC, National Academy Press, 224–249, 1986.

Brody, B.: *Life and Death Decision Making.* New York, Oxford, 1988.

Brown, M.T.: *Working Ethics.* San Francisco, Jossey-Bass, 1990.

Buie, J.: Given lemons, they make lemonade. *APA Monitor, 20,* 1989.

Calabresi, G. and Bobbitt, P.: *Tragic Choices.* New York, Norton, 1978.

Callahan, D.: Modernizing mortality: Medical progress and the good society. *Hastings Center Report,* 20:28–32, 1990b.

Childress, J.H.: *Who Should Decide?: Paternalism in Health Care.* New York, Oxford, 1982.

Childress, J.H.: The place of autonomy in bioethics. *Hastings Center Report, 20:*12–17, 1990.

Coles, R.: The end of the affair. *Katallagete:* Be Reconciled, *4:*46–58, 1972.

Dougherty, C.J.: Ethical perspectives on prospective payment. *Hastings Center Report, 19:*5–11, 1989.

Dyer, A.R.: *Ethics and Psychiatry.* Washington, D.C., American Psychiatric Press, 1988.

Estes, C.L.: *The Aging Enterprise.* San Francisco, Jossey-Bass, 1979.

Faden, R.R. and Beauchamp, T.L.: *A History and Theory of Informed Consent.* New York, Oxford, 1986.

Fein, R.: For profits: A look at the bottom line. *Journal of Public Health Policy, 11:*49–61, 1990.

Field, M.F. and Gray, B.H.: Should we regulate "Utilization Management?" *Health Affairs, 8:*103–112, 1989.

Freidson, E.: *Professional Dominance.* Chicago, Aldine, 1970.

Fuchs, V.R.: *Who Shall Live?* New York, Basic Books, 1974.

Gray, B.H. (Ed.): *For-Profit Enterprise in Health Care.* Institute of Medicine, Washington, D.C., National Academy Press, 1986.

Gray, B.H. and Field, M. F. (Eds.): *Controlling Costs and Changing Patient Care? The Role of Utilization Management.* Institute of Medicine, Washington, D.C., National Academy Press, 1989.

Grossman, M.: Insurance reports as a threat to confidentiality. *American Journal of Psychiatry, 128:*96–100, 1971.

Jonsen, A.R., Seigler, M. and Winslade, W.J.: *Clinical Ethics,* 3rd Ed. New York, Macmillan, 1986.

Katz, J.: *The Silent World of Doctor and Patient.* New York, Free Press, 1984.

Keith-Spiegel, P. and Koocher, G.P.: *Ethics in Psychology.* New York, Random, 1985.

Kleinman, A.: *The Illness Narratives.* New York, Basic Books, 1988.

Kongstvedt, P.R. (Ed.): *The Managed Health Care Handbook.* Rockville, MD, Aspen, 1989.

Larkin, H.: Managed mental health care moves inpatients out. *Hospitals,* 1989.

Levine, M.: *Psychiatry and Ethics.* New York, Braziller, 1972.

McKinley, J. B. and Arches, J.: Toward the proletarianization of physicians. *International Journal of Health Services, 15:*161–195, 1985.

McKinley, J. and Stoeckle, J.: Corporatization and the social transformation of doctoring. *International Journal of Health Services,* 18:191–205, 1988. Reprinted in Conrad, P. and Kern, R. (Eds.): *The Sociology of Health and Illness,* 3rd ed. New York, St. Martin's Press, 1990.

Monahan, J. (Ed.): *Who Is The Client: The Ethics of Psychological Intervention in the Criminal Justice System.* Washington, DC, American Psychological Association, 1980.

Relman, A.S.: The new medical-industrial complex. *New England Journal of Medicine, 303:*963–970, 1980.

Relman, A.S. and Reinhardt, U.: An exchange on for-profit health care. In Gray, B.H. (Ed.).: *For-Profit Enterprise in Health Care.* Institute of Medicine, Washington, D.C., National Academy Press, 1986.

Sabin, J.E.: Psychiatrists face tough ethical questions in managed care settings. *The Psychiatric Times,* 1989.

Shelp, E.E. (Ed.): *Justice and Health Care.* Boston, Reidel, 1981.

Starr, P.: *The Social Transformation of American Medicine.* New York, Basic Books, 1982.

Staver, S.: Employers turning to managed mental health care. *American Medical News, 1:*13–14, 1989.

Van Hoose, W.H. and Kottler, J.A.: *Ethical and Legal Issues in Counseling and Psychotherapy,* 2nd ed. San Francisco, Jossey-Bass, 1985.

Veatch, R.M. and Branson, R. (Eds.): *Ethics and Health Policy.* Cambridge, MA, Ballinger, 1976.

Vladeck, B.C.: The market vs. regulation: the case for regulation. *Milbank Memorial Fund Quarterly, 59:*209–223, 1981.

Wojcik, J.: *Muted Consent.* West Lafayette, IN, Purdue University Press, 1978.

Chapter 13

MANAGED MENTAL HEALTH: KEY LEGAL ISSUES

J. Peter Rich

T his chapter provides an overview of the legal issues affecting managed mental health, with a focus on those at the cutting edge. There are many such, ranging from the liability of managed mental health entities for discharging patients who then harm themselves or others, to antitrust and tax law issues. Their importance is likely to grow as cost containment pressures compel payors to deal with the increasing cost of mental disorders and substance abuse.[1]

The chapter first examines the federal and state regulatory environment in which the managed care industry and mental health professionals work. Next, it addresses various legal issues confronting certain types of provider-controlled managed care entities. Finally, areas of potential legal liability are examined; some of these are specific to mental health, at least in their application, while others apply to managed care generally.

Government Regulation of Health Maintenance Organizations

In response to unprecedented health care cost inflation, health maintenance organizations (HMOs) emerged by the late 1970s as a major alternative to traditional indemnity insurance programs that provided no incentives to control utilization. Although managed care entities had existed since the mid-1940s, it was only in the 1970s that managed care in the form of the HMO emerged as a principal means of restraining health care costs. The emergence of HMOs was fostered by the federal Act of 1980 (42 U.S.C., section 330e et seq.) that offered federal financial support in the form of grants and low-cost loans to HMOs that met certain standards.

---

1. The author would like to acknowledge the assistance of his associates at McDermott, Will & Emery, Kandy F. Waldie and Peter J. Martin, in the preparation of this chapter.

HMOs are regulated primarily at the state level—all states require licensure. Most of them regulate HMOs under specific enabling statutes, with licensing and oversight authority in the hands of the state's insurance regulators. In others, regulation of the health delivery function of the HMO (quality assurance, accessibility to care, etc.) is delegated to the state health department or, in the case of California, for example, to the Department of Corporations.

State regulatory concerns have focused on fiscal soundness and the quality of care, by overseeing the adequacy of provider networks and quality assurance standards. Because HMOs are subject to state insurance regulation, they generally are required to meet the benefit mandates imposed on health insurers. Twenty-eight states require some form of mental health benefit; 22 require coverage for drug abuse services, and 40 require alcoholism benefits (BCBSA Survey, 1989). The United States has ruled that these state mandated benefit laws are not preempted by the Employee Retirement Income Security Act of 1974 ("ERISA").[2,3]

Single-Service HMOs

The single-service HMO, such as mental health or dental, is one form that has not yet been closely regulated. In some states, the HMO enabling statute provides for the licensure and operation of HMOs that do not provide a comprehensive range of services. Mental health plans are rarely recognized. California has been at the forefront of such single-service plans; as of early 1990, there were several licensed mental health HMOs and others pending licensure. California has also taken the lead in prohibiting the operation of what the regulators deem to be unlicensed mental health plans—those providing such services as case management, coordination and management of provider networks, and employee assistance programs. Although the wording of the HMO enabling laws in many states seem to allow such entities to be regulated, few states other than California have thus far taken such a restrictive approach. It would be unwise, however, for such unlicensed programs outside California to view this situation with complacency. California's HMO regulators are leaders in the national association and historically have exerted significant influence upon trends in state HMO regulation across

---

2. *Metropolitan Life Insurance Co.* vs. *Massachusetts,* 471 U.S. 724, 105 S. Ct. 2380 (1985).

3. ERISA is the federal law that regulates self-funded pension and welfare benefit plans established by employers or employee organizations.

the country. Furthermore, the National Association of Insurance Commissioners ("NAIC") has written a "Prepaid Limited Health Service Organization Model Act," and both Illinois and Nebraska have adopted statutes closely following this model.

OTHER REGULATORY ISSUES

Employee Assistance Programs

One employer response to burgeoning mental health and substance abuse costs for their employees has been the employee assistance program ("EAP"). Of 220 employers surveyed by Coopers and Lybrand, 147 had considered implementing an EAP and 115 had one in place. Some EAPs are operated internally, using personnel employed by the company; others are provided through contracts with outside vendors. A number of managed care entities offer EAPs and some EAP firms are adding managed mental health programs. A growing number of EAPs have obtained an HMO license so that they may offer a full range of mental health and substance abuse services on a capitated basis.

If an employer provides EAP services solely through its own employees, the EAP is generally not subject to state regulation because of the ERISA preemption. ERISA preemption applies only to state insurance laws, however, and does not shelter such employers from malpractice or other lawsuits based upon the misconduct of employees providing EAP services. A number of suits, for example, have been brought against employers of psychotherapists for sexual misconduct. Courts have rendered conflicting rulings on whether an employer operating an in-house EAP program can be liable for such conduct (Medical Liability Reporter, 1989).

EAPs may be subject to state regulation if they are established through contracts with outside providers who are at financial risk for providing the EAP services. In California, for example, the HMO statute regulates any entity that provides or arranges for health care services in return for a prepaid or periodic charge, including EAPs. A very limited regulatory exemption from California HMO licensure applies to EAPs that provide no more than three assessment and referral visits per employee in any six-month period. Thus, in California, if an outside EAP contractor bears the financial risk of providing services beyond the limited EAP exemption, no matter how minimal the risk may be, it must be licensed as an HMO.

Professional Licensure

Insuring that practitioners adhere to state licensure requirements and limit their activities to the scope of their licenses is likely to become an increasingly important quality assurance issue for managed mental health entities. All states require psychiatrists to be licensed physicians with specialized psychiatric training. Licensure requirements of other mental health practitioners—from psychologists to social workers to professional counselors—vary widely from state to state. While almost all require psychologists to be licensed, approximately 18 states have enacted social worker licensure statutes, and six require a license for professional counselors, including addiction counselors. In some states, use of such allied mental health professionals is part of mandated benefits statutes: health insurance laws require the inclusion of professional counselor services in four states (California, Montana, New Hampshire and Virginia), while 14 states now require insurers to cover social workers.

Confidentiality of Patient Records

Patient record confidentiality statutes exist in most states, as do laws generally protecting the confidentiality of communications between patients and physicians. These laws are of particular importance in managed care, which is dependent upon the continuous and open sharing of information about patients. Mental health information is protected by the most restrictive state and federal confidentiality statutes, matched or surpassed only by those dealing with AIDS.

Many states have statutes specifically protecting the confidentiality of the medical records of psychiatric patients. These statutes, however, generally permit third-party payors to inspect patient records in the normal course of determining eligibility or entitlement to benefits. They also allow access to such records for good-faith application of peer review procedures.

Similar state statutes often govern the confidentiality of substance abuse records. Federal statutes and regulations prohibit disclosure of identifying information on patients diagnosed or treated for substance abuse in a federally-assisted treatment program. Under the federal law, such a program is defined as any person or organization that provides alcohol or drug abuse diagnosis, treatment or referral for treatment and that (1) receives any funds from the federal government, (2) is Medicare certified, (3) is tax exempt or is allowed tax deductions for contributions, or (4) is conducted directly by the federal, state or local government. These regulations, however, also permit the copying or removal of such records for "audit and evaluation" activities performed by a third-party payor or a peer review organization conducting utilization or quality control reviews; provided that the third-party payor or peer review organization agrees in writing (1) not to redisclose the information received to any other person, (2) to destroy, upon completion of the review, all information that would identify a patient, (3) to maintain the information in a locked or secure place, and (4) to adopt written procedures for regulating the use of the records.

It does not appear that confidentiality requirements have hindered managed mental health firms, although conflicts may increase as utilization controls become stricter, and legislatures respond to perceived abuses by employers and managed care entities.

Preferred Provider Organizations

The most significant recent trend in the managed care field has been the development of preferred provider organizations (PPOs). One estimate is that, by the end of 1988, 36 million people had access to PPOs (Fox, 1990). Under contractual arrangement, preferred providers discount their fees and, in return, health benefit plans give their enrollees financial incentives to use the PPO. For example, a particular service might have a $500 deductible and a 10% coinsurance obligation if provided by a member of a PPO; the same service might involve a $1,000–$1,500 deductible and a 20% or higher coinsurance obligation if the enrollee goes outside of the PPO network.

PPOs are most often sponsored by Blue Cross-Blue Shield plans, insurance companies, self-insured employers and union trusts, who contract either directly or through intermediaries with groups of physicians, hospitals and other providers. Employers or union trusts with self-insured plans typically contract with a third party administrator (TPA) to administer their plans. Legally, a TPA may be an insurance company that provides administrative services only, or it may be a separately licensed TPA company. TPAs and PPOs are subject to a diverse set of regulatory requirements, but not to the extent of HMOs. Many states have taken a relatively laissez-faire attitude toward PPOs. Moreover, PPOs sponsored by self-insured employers and union trusts are largely exempt from any state regulation under ERISA (Rolph, 1986).

Unlike HMOs, PPOs are not (and legally often cannot be, unless they have their own HMO license) paid on either a salaried or capitation basis[4]; rather they are paid a discounted fee-for-service. Consequently, PPO providers are not at risk for overutilization. Moreover, PPO enrollees are free to choose any health care provider without giving up all or most of their benefit coverage; instead they pay a significant but generally manageable financial penalty for going outside the PPO. In these ways, the PPO resembles traditional fee-for-service health care. However, PPOs are increasingly subjecting their participating providers and enrollees to various forms of utilization review (UR) that were first developed by HMOs and represent a key element of managed care.

The extent of such review by a PPO was recently challenged by several Ohio psychiatrists and patients. In this case, the state of Ohio contracted with a managed care firm to manage the State's mental health and substance abuse insurance program. The plaintiffs charged that the firm's requirements that care be reviewed every three sessions to determine medical necessity and that patients under existing care switch to its providers were too restrictive.

Recently, PPOs have begun to take on another HMO characteristic; closed provider panels. Known as "exclusive provider organizations" (EPOs) or exclusive provider arrangement (EPAs), or sometimes as generic HMOs, these plans offer little or no coverage for non-emergency out-of-panel services. They are one of the fastest growing forms of managed care.

There is essentially no federal regulation of PPOs as such. The 1988 amendments to the HMO statute permit federally-qualified HMOs to offer their enrollees a "wrap-around" HMO–PPO product, sometimes called a "point-of-service" option because the enrollee can choose at the time of needed medical treatment whether to use an HMO or PPO. The closest PPO analogue to federal qualification currently available is an accreditation program recently initiated by the American Association of Preferred Provider Organizations. So far, only one PPO has undergone an accreditation survey (Managed HealthCare, 1989).

---

4. For example, California and many other states follow this regulatory approach. Moreover, the Maryland Attorney General recently ruled that such an arrangement required an HMO license.

State Regulation

State regulation of PPOs is much less prevalent than for HMOs. Through 1989, at least 20 states had passed PPO enabling acts applicable to PPOs affiliated with commercial insurance companies and the Blues. Many states, however, prohibit health insurers from restricting an insured's freedom to choose a health care provider. These so-called "freedom of choice" statutes exist in approximately 33 jurisdictions and in those, extreme measures to "channel" enrollees into insurer PPOs may be interpreted as interfering with freedom of choice. In the EPO, for example, enrollees are permitted to receive care only from the designated panel. Freedom of choice statutes may prohibit such "lock-ins." As discussed below, however, ERISA preemption generally allows self-insured employers and union trust funds to ignore these state restrictions.

Another type of state PPO regulation takes the form of anti-discrimination statutes. These generally prohibit insurance companies from unfairly discriminating between individuals in the same risk class as to the amount of premium or rates charged. Almost every state has an anti-discrimination statute in its insurance laws. PPOs that require enrollees to pay more for out-of-network services, may find these arrangements to violate such statutes. Almost all anti-discrimination statutes, however, prohibit only "unfair" discrimination. This typically means that out-of-network providers must be reimbursed an amount at least equal to 75–85% of the PPO rate. To the extent that benefit differentials really preserve enrollees' freedom to use out-of-network providers (albeit at a higher cost), this might not be defined as unfair.

A few states have enacted "any willing provider" statutes. These generally require that all providers meeting certain objective criteria be entitled to reimbursement for services they render to enrollees. Depending on how restrictive the criteria are, such statutes may significantly impede a PPO's efforts to contract only with certain providers on the basis of quality of care or for purposes of tailoring the PPO to particular market conditions.

Under ERISA, PPOs sponsored by self-insured employers or union trusts can largely escape both state insurance and HMO regulation. Because a self-funded PPO is considered an employee benefit plan rather than an insurance company, it is subject to ERISA provisions regarding minimum participation, funding and vesting standards and certain limits on employee contributions and benefits. These are far less onerous than state HMO and PPO laws. The scope of the ERISA preemption, however, remains uncertain, although the recent trend has been for the courts to interpret it broadly. In this regard, recent federal case law suggests that where a self-funded PPO contracts with an insurance company for coverage of extraordinary medical expenses—so-called "stop-loss" insurance—it has, in effect, become an insurance company and thus loses the benefits of ERISA preemption.[5] The same limitations on ERISA may well allow HMO regulators to retain jurisdiction over brokers and providers who contract with self-insured employers on a capitated basis. As self-insured plans strive to implement creative new managed care arrangements that include capitation but attempt to avoid the "middle-man's profit" by eschewing HMOs, this issue of ERISA preemption is likely to be hotly contested in the federal courts.

PROVIDER–CONTROLLED NETWORKS AND ANTITRUST LIABILITY

Providers of mental health and substance abuse services who want to participate in managed care have increasingly turned to the independent practice association (IPA). An IPA enters into discounted fee-for-service or capitated contracts with providers. In the managed care industry, IPAs have been at the leading edge of growth and innovation: since 1984, the IPA model has grown from 40% to over 60% of all HMOs (*Modern Healthcare,* 1989). In part, this growth is due to their willingness to assume a portion of the risk of providing care to health plan enrollees. This trend is apparent in mental health as well. Provider risk-sharing is seen as one of the means by which managed mental health can achieve more efficient care (*Managed Care Outlook,* 1989). With the rise in single specialty HMOs has come a concomitant trend toward single service IPAs, including those devoted exclusively to mental health.

The formation of an IPA raises certain legal and organizational issues, whether or not it is single specialty. Perhaps the most sensitive and complex of these arises in response to Section 414(m) of the Internal Revenue Code. While this section was intended to apply to perceived abuses by professionals in the use of tax-advantaged pension plans, its scope includes IPAs. If an IPA and one or more professional corporations,

---

5. Michigan United Food vs. Baerwaldt, 767 F.2d 308 (6th Cir. 1985), cert. denied 474 U.S. 1059, 106 S. Ct. 801 (1986).

medical groups, partnerships or individual physicians are deemed to constitute an "affiliated service group," they will all be treated as a single employer for purposes of determining whether the retirement plan of any member of the affiliated service group complies with applicable anti-discrimination, eligibility, vesting contribution and benefit limit requirements. An IPA may be deemed an affiliated service group, even if it has no employees, if it has one or more owners (shareholders or corporate members) or "highly compensated employees" who meet certain income requirements. If the affiliated service group rules are applied to an IPA and its owners or highly compensated employees, the tax-preferred status of their retirement plans would be jeopardized. This could result in the imposition of a substantial tax liability on those owners, even if the IPA itself had no pension plan.

Given this risk, an IPA should be organized either with no owners, no owners who have pension plans, or as a one-shareholder professional corporation. Theoretically, IPA owners could be limited to persons with pension plans that are "comparable" to the IPA's pension plan under IRS rules, but this is likely to be impractical. Alternatively, the owners could decide to run this risk after it has been fully disclosed to them, since there has not yet been any reported cases of an IPA and its owners suffering pension plan disqualification.

Other legal requirements constrain the choice of the IPA corporate form. The use of a business corporation format is barred by most states that have "corporate practice of medicine statutes." These require that medical services be rendered only by licensed persons, individually or in medical groups, and by professional corporations. The fact that partnership laws in almost all states make the partners jointly and severally liable for the actions of the partnership make this type of structure unattractive to the IPA.

An IPA organized as a professional corporation avoids the "corporate practice of medicine" prohibition, limits the liability of the shareholders, and, if the shareholders and officers do not have their own pension plans or stay below certain stock ownership and income thresholds, can reduce the risk under the affiliated service group rules. If the professional corporation is formed with only one shareholder, issues may arise regarding that shareholder's control of the corporation and its profits.

Antitrust Liability

The spectre of antitrust liability lends special importance to carefully structuring an IPA with regard to selection of participants and establishment of professional fees. Antitrust liability is basically founded on two federal laws, the Sherman and the Clayton Acts. The Sherman Act prohibits conspiracies in restraint of trade and bars monopolization and attempts to monopolize. The Clayton Act forbids tie-ins and exclusive contracts and governs certain mergers and acquisitions. There are other antitrust-related statutes,[6] but anti-trust issues in the managed care field usually focus on these two.

Conspiracy liability requires an agreement in or affecting interstate commerce between two economically distinct parties that unreasonably restrain trade. Thus, if the parties to an agreement are sufficiently integrated into one entity, no conspiracy is possible. Also, a restraint of trade agreement among entities in competition with each other (so-called "horizontal" restraints) runs a greater risk of violating the antitrust laws than do agreements among entities at different levels of distribution, such as agreements between a manufacturer and a dealer (so-called "vertical" restraints). Thus, a price-fixing agreement among competitors may be condemned as an anti-competitive restraint of trade. The classic example of such price fixing was found to be unlawful in *Arizona* vs. *Maricopa County Medical Society,* where the United States Supreme Court held it was "per se" illegal for physicians to adopt a maximum fee schedule through a provider-controlled organization.

There are three general approaches to minimizing the risk that an IPA will be found guilty of horizontal price fixing in setting professional fees. First, the IPA might function merely as a "conduit" or "messenger" of price information to its participating practitioners, negotiating with third parties only on non-price contract terms, such as utilization review/quality assurance or billing practices. Each physician would then separately agree to the proposed rates or attempt to negotiate different ones. This approach, while safest from an antitrust perspective, is very time consuming, unwieldly, and thus not favored by providers or payors.

Second, and probably best, an IPA could adopt a blended professional fee schedule, preferably recommended by an independent third party, or sign third-party payor agreements proposing such a fee schedule, so

---

6. E.g., The Federal Trade Commission Act and The Robinson-Patman Act.

long as each individual practitioner has a period of time (e.g., 10 days) within which to "opt out" of this arrangement. This approach is most popular among start-up IPAs that are not yet ready to accept risk-sharing arrangements but wish to negotiate professional fees collectively with third-party payors. While not entirely free of risk, this approach should withstand a price-fixing challenge, particularly when combined with a collective agreement not to balance bill enrollees, to take assignment where required, to accept utilization review restrictions, and to follow other dictates of the IPA as well as any third-party payor contracts. Of course, the IPA should also be pro-competitive and should represent no more than 50–60% of the practitioners in the applicable service area, (or 20%–30% if the IPA is the exclusive contracting entity for those practitioners), in order to minimize antitrust risks.

Third, IPA physicians may agree among themselves as to fees so long as the IPA is a legitimate, "integrated" joint venture, as demonstrated by significant financial contributions or more commonly, substantial risk sharing. The joint venture approach shields the IPA from antitrust liability on the theory that a new product is being offered as to which price requirements are integral. It is crucial that the practitioners be at risk if the IPA is unable to operate within its budget.[7] At a minimum, they should be subject to some withhold of their professional fees, to be paid only if utilization management and other targets have been met, individually and collectively.

Another area of potential antitrust liability has to do with the selection of participants. This can run afoul of the prohibition in the Sherman Act of "group boycotts." In general, liability of this type arises only if the provider-controlled organization which denies participation has significant market power or an anti-competitive purpose. It may also arise if the organization has a dominant share of local providers and excludes all who affiliate with other organizations.

IPAs commonly require staff membership at one or more local hospitals for those seeking to participate in it. Particularly if the IPA has or is likely to obtain significant market power, it should take steps to insure that its credentialing process incorporates legitimate business and quality-of-care criteria. Additionally, the IPA should follow its credentialing

---

7. Where a group of ophthalmologists contributed $10,000 and participated in a capitation program for some services, the FTC found "significant integration among . . . physician shareholders" where the physicians "made capital contributions and assumed a degree of risk and created a product none of them could produce alone." (Unpublished FTC advisory note.)

procedures in every case. In a currently-pending action in the U.S. District Court for the Northern District of New York (*Capital Imaging Associates, P.D.* vs. *Mohawk Valley Medical Associates, Inc.*), the court agreed to hear the plaintiff's claim of a conspiracy to exclude him from IPA membership. The IPA allegedly had refused to send the plaintiff a membership application upon his request, in contravention of the IPA's credentialing procedure. The risk here is that the refusal to send an application might be ruled a denial motivated by anti-competitive purposes. An IPA that consistently follows its credentialing procedures can more easily document its refusal to deal with a particular provider for legitimate reasons.

Not only should an IPA consistently follow its credentialing procedures, but the criteria for participation should be such as to identify quality, cost-effective providers. An IPA should set certain objective standards for participating and solicit information from applicants in order to evaluate their qualifications. The criteria could be based upon such factors as utilization patterns, thoroughness and timeliness in completing medical records, board certification or eligibility, fee level, willingness to participate in committee work, referral patterns, attitude toward peer review, and general reputation.

It is essential that the criteria established be reasonably related to the objectives of the IPA and uniformly applied to all applicants. Deficiencies in these areas could result in lawsuits brought by excluded or expelled providers alleging that the IPA's actions were the product of anti-competitive or other unlawful motives. There is a lesser risk of liability if a practitioner is excluded at the outset, rather than expelled.

A recent federal court decision illustrates some of the issues described above. In the case of *Hassan* vs. *Independent Practice Association, P.C.*, two allergists alleged, among other things, that an IPA maximum fee schedule set fees below competitive levels and drove them out of the market. The IPA received monthly capitation payments from an HMO that were subject to an approximate 12% risk withhold, and paid its members according to a fee schedule. The court found that the fee schedule was a necessary part of a legitimate joint venture: it was part of a risk-sharing program by physicians participating in the IPA. The court also characterized the IPA fee setting as a means of distributing revenue from the HMO to IPA members, not as an illegal price-fixing scheme.

The *Hassan* plaintiffs also alleged that the IPA's expulsion of them was an illegal boycott. The court found that the expulsion was pursuant to an

IPA policy that limited the use of certain diagnostic tests. This policy was based on cost-containment objectives with the court found to be pro-competitive.

Another antitrust issue related to the selection of practitioners is the potential risk of liability for monopolization under the Sherman Act. As an IPA grows, so does the importance of attending to this risk. If the IPA requires that practitioners participate on an exclusive basis, they can no longer compete with each other. If they represent a sufficiently large share of the providers in the relevant geographic area, the exclusive arrangement might be deemed an unreasonable restraint on competition. A useful rule of thumb for exclusive contracting is 20% to 30% of the practitioners in the area. On the other hand, non-exclusive contracts representing up to 50% to 60% of them pose no antitrust problems.

Peer Review Activities

A final point regarding antitrust liability concerns the possible availability of limited immunity from liability for damages under antitrust and other federal and state laws under the Health Care Quality Improvement Act of 1986 ("the act"). Assuming that IPAs fall within the terms of the act as a "group medical practice" (which while undefined appears to apply to IPAs), they may qualify for the act's "safe harbor" for its credentialing and peer review activities. If an IPA chooses to contract with a separate entity to perform credentialing and other peer review services, it might not fall within the terms of the act. If an IPA performs these functions itself, it must insure that its peer review process is fair and reasonable, although as a legal matter the IPA is not obligated to provide a "fair hearing" as required of hospitals or even "notice and an opportunity to be heard," unless required by state law.

Some states have enacted legislation that requires IPAs to provide notice, hearing and appeal rights to physicians in addition to the rights set forth in the act. California, for example, recently enacted new legislation that mandates certain notice and hearing rights for physicians and others who are subject to certain medical disciplinary peer review actions by medical groups and IPAs. Moreover, California law requires IPAs and other groups to notify the state's medical board of certain medical disciplinary action taken against a physician by an IPA.

MANAGED MENTAL HEALTH LIABILITY ISSUES

Provider Credentialing and Peer Review Liability

HMOs and other managed care organizations have been held liable for the malpractice of providers associated with them in a number of circumstances and under a variety of legal theories. The factual scenarios and legal principles relevant to HMOs and their practitioners generally apply to mental health practitioners.

The legal theory that an employer is vicariously liable for the acts or omissions of his employees, the doctrine of respondeat superior, has been applied to hospitals since early in this century. Lately, the same doctrine has been extended to HMOs. In the case of *Sloan* vs. *Metropolitan Health Council of Indianapolis, Inc.*, the health plan held itself out to the public as the employer of the physicians and treated its contracted physicians as employees in terms of salary, taxes, fringe benefits and in requiring the plan's consent for practice elsewhere. The court found that these facts supported the existence of an agency or employer-employee relationship, and therefore the plan's vicarious liability for the malpractice of its contracting physicians. Similarly, in the case of *Schleier* vs. *Kaiser Foundation Health Plan*, a federal appeals court ruled that a staff-model HMO (i.e., the HMO employs the physician) could be held liable for the acts of a consulting cardiologist who was an independent contractor of the HMO. The consultant, who was called into the case by a Kaiser primary care physician (PCP), misdiagnosed the patient's condition and he later died of a heart attack. Applying District of Columbia law, the court found that Kaiser could be held vicariously liable for the consultant's malpractice because Kaiser selected and engaged the consultant, could discharge him, controlled his actions through the authority exercised by Kaiser's PCP, and because the consultant's efforts were part of Kaiser's regular business.

Another theory of legal liability, that of "ostensible agency," holds that when an entity represents to a third party that a non-employee is in fact an agent of the entity, it may be liable for the non-employee's actions. This theory was applied to an HMO in the case of *Boyd* vs. *Albert Einstein Medical Center*, where the HMO advertised that its providers were competent and utilized a PCP "gatekeeper" system whereby the provision of specialist care required authorization by the PCP. The plaintiff was permitted by the court to proceed with her ostensible agency claim because of the HMO's representations and because the restriction on access to specialist medical care represented by the gatekeeper system may have led the patient to refrain from seeing a specialist to obtain needed care. Although the *Boyd* case has not yet been decided, this case is important in that the court held that the HMO *could* be held liable if certain facts were established by the plaintiff.

Under a third theory of liability, an HMO and other managed care organization may be found liable for the negligent selection of one of its providers. The theory of "corporate negligence" was applied to an HMO for the first time in the case of *Harrell* vs. *Total Health Care,* where it was found that the HMO failed to conduct a reasonable investigation into a specialist physician's competence. The court ruled that the HMO had a duty to adequately credential its providers; this duty arose because of the HMO's control over its enrollees' choice of provider. The court found that the HMO breached this duty by failing to make any investigation beyond inquiring as to professional licensure, hospital privileges and narcotics licensure. The HMO consequently could be held directly liable for the specialist's negligence in treating an HMO enrollee. Although the Missouri Supreme Court later ruled that a statute immunizing the HMO from this liability was constitutional, the *Harrell* case supports the principle of HMO corporate liability for negligent selection of physicians.

In general, the lessons of the body of HMO case law apply to managed mental health entities: managed care control over providers can lead to liability for their mistakes. Some of the mechanisms used by managed care systems to assure quality, such as provider credentialing or gatekeeper authorization of services, must be utilized carefully because when a plan undertakes to assure quality care it also is at risk for liability when quality care is not delivered. For this reason, effective credentialing and peer review are very important.

Utilization Review Decisions

Perhaps the most widely discussed area of liability for managed care malpractice is that of utilization review (UR) or utilization management (UM). These terms refer, in general, to efforts to manage the use of health care resources in a cost-effective manner while maintaining quality of care. The traditionally close connection between utilization review and quality assurance (QA) is reflected in the fact that they are often discussed together. Utilization management includes such elements as prospective review of non-emergency hospital admissions and of clinical procedures and tests through pre-admission certification, assigned inpatient lengths of stay and second opinions. Other mechanisms are concurrent review, retrospective chart audits, and case management systems.

Wickline vs. *California* was the first significant case in the area of managed care liability for UR/QA decisions. In that case the court held that an HMO or PPO may be held liable for utilization management decisions resulting from defects in the design or implementation of a utilization review program. Briefly, the facts in *Wickline* were that a California physician who requested an eight-day hospital extension for a MediCal (Medicaid) patient, acquiesced in a physician advisor's approval of a four-day extension instead. Medical complications ensued, allegedly due to the shortened hospital stay, and the patient sued the state of California, arguing that MediCal's cost-containment mechanism caused a premature hospital discharge. The California Court of Appeals reversed the jury's award of $500,000 to the plaintiff on the grounds that the treating physician never protested the extension denial, so MediCal had no opportunity to override his decision. However, the court issued this warning:

> Third-party payors can be held legally accountable when medically inappropriate decisions result from defects in the design or implementation of cost containment mechanisms as, for example, when appeals made on a patient's behalf for medical or hospital care are arbitrarily ignored or unreasonably disregarded or overridden.

In the case of *Sarchett* vs. *Blue Shield of California,* an insurer's failure to inform a subscriber of his right to appeal a denial of hospital stay led to liability for the plan. In the *Sarchett* case, Blue Shield of California's continuous failure to tell the subscriber of his appeal rights while repeatedly denying the subscriber's claim was held to be designed to mislead subscribers into forfeiting their contractual rights. Thus, a health plan may be required to inform enrollees of their review and appeal rights whenever benefits are denied.

A related area of potential utilization management liability is that of medical necessity determinations. Another California case (*Hughes* vs. *Blue Cross of Northern California*) dealt with a Blue Cross plan's denial of hospital benefits to a subscriber on the ground that a lower level of care was medically appropriate. An appellate court found that this decision was based on a medical necessity standard at significant variance with community standards and concluded that good faith required use of the community standard.[8]

Utilization management as applied to mental health professionals was recently discussed in a Michigan case, *Varol* vs. *Blue Cross and Blue Shield of Michigan,* in which the court dismissed claims by psychiatrist plaintiffs challenging UR under state law; the court held that ERISA preempted their claims. The court chose, however, to discuss the "actual merits" of the allegation that the triple-option health plan's pre-authorization requirement for psychiatric care interfered with the psychiatrists' medical judgment. The managed psychiatric care program called for pre-authorization by health plan employees and review by a psychiatrist; if the proposed treatment plan was not approved, the treating psychiatrist could proceed with the plan but the health plan would pay only 80% of his fee and the psychiatrist would then have to obtain the remaining 20% from the patient. The court criticized the plaintiff psychiatrists for advancing the theory that this pre-authorization program would have any effect on their ethical and legal obligation to provide appropriate treatment.

A recent California case also addressed utilization management in the mental health field, and in so doing, sharply criticized the language in the *Wickline* decision as being "overbroad." In the case of *Wilson* vs. *Blue Cross of Southern California,* Wilson, a Blue Cross beneficiary, was admitted to a hospital suffering from major depression, drug dependency and anorexia. The Blue Cross contract provided for mental health benefits of 30 days. After 10 days in the hospital, Wilson was told that Blue Cross would not pay for further hospital care. Wilson's physician determined that he needed three to four weeks of inpatient care. As Wilson had no money available to pay for further care, he was discharged. Three weeks later he committed suicide. Western Medical Review, the entity that made the utilization review decision, claimed that the principles enumerated in *Wickline* shielded it from liability. The *Wilson* court rejected this argument on the grounds that the *Wickline* language relied upon was dicta and misstated tort law principles on joint liability. Because there was a material factual question whether the utilization review decision to no longer pay for Wilson's hospitalization was a substantial factor in

---

8. It should be noted that under Oregon law, a mental health utilization review program is not limited to denials of claims for lack of medical necessity: if a lower level of care would have been medically appropriate, the utilization review process can approve payment appropriate to the lower level of care.

causing Wilson's suicide, the appellate court reversed the trial court's grant of Western Medical Review's motion for summary judgment.

The *Wilson* case is significant in that it restricts the *Wickline* case to its facts, specific to the California Medicaid program. The *Wilson* court ruled as irrelevant the fact that Wilson's treating physician never appealed the utilization review decision since there was no evidence that the physician could have, or knew he could have, appealed, nor that an appeal would have been successful. The court held that "the availability of an avenue of appeal fails to prove as a matter of law that [Wilson's] demise was unrelated to his denial of benefits." *Wilson* rejected the parts of *Wickline* that protected payors and other entities doing utilization review. Regardless of whether the treating physician was negligent, the payor may be liable if its utilization review decision was a "substantial factor" in causing harm to the beneficiary. Since *Wilson* (and *Wickline*) involved individual insurance coverage, it is unclear whether they would apply to group insurance plans.

This case law suggests that in utilization management, the treating practitioner's ultimate responsibility for decision-making may be subject to an exception, or may be shared, where a managed care entity's utilization management mechanism does not or cannot adequately accommodate the practitioner's clinical judgment. Utilization management mechanisms must be designed and implemented competently, and must result in clinically defensible decisions (Blum, 1989). Payors can strive to minimize their exposure in this area by using only professional personnel and state of the art systems, by not denying coverage if there is any doubt, and making sure that all UM decisions are consistent with both community medical standards and plan criteria. How to accomplish these goals in the mental health arena, as well as in other medical fields, and still accomplish cost containment objectives, is and will remain a difficult problem for some time.

Risk Sharing and Restrictive Referrals

Another cost-containment device widely used in managed care is the use of financial incentives to encourage cost-effective services. These incentives often take the form of risk-sharing by providers in which a portion of their reimbursement is withheld, to be used at year end to cover any deficits, or to be distributed. Only a few court cases have been filed about the use of such arrangements. As the impetus for constraining the rising costs of mental health and substance abuse increases, the use of risk-sharing mechanisms by managed care entities is likely to increase.

In the case of *Pulvers* vs. *Kaiser Foundation Health Plan*, the plaintiff claimed that the plan's financial arrangements caused its physicians not to diagnose a disease because the physicians had financial incentives to limit tests and treatment. The court rejected this claim, noting that incentive arrangements are recommended by professional organizations and required by the federal HMO Act.

Despite the *Pulvers* decision, other cases have been filed presenting similar arguments. A class action filed against the U.S. Healthcare HMO (*Teti* vs. *U.S. Healthcare, Inc.*) by some of its members, challenged the physician fee withhold and incentive arrangements. The plaintiffs claimed that these arrangements rendered the care to be of lesser quality than the HMO represented in its marketing materials. The dismissal of this action was recently affirmed on appeal. The case of *Bush* vs. *Dake*, recently dismissed by the court, was based on the claim that the HMOs gatekeeper system, capitation and risk pool arrangements with a group practice caused undue delay in the diagnosis of the plaintiff's cancer. In this case, the trial court held that the plaintiff may have stated a viable theory of liability in arguing that the HMOs payment arrangements proximately caused her injuries.

In Oregon, a group of psychologists recently filed suit against an HMO that hired a managed mental health company to manage and provide the HMOs mental health benefits (Managed Health Care, 1989). Under the terms of the HMOs contract, its enrollees must use the panel of providers of the managed mental health company, unless that panel lacks the appropriate expertise. The company also provides pre-authorization and concurrent review of mental health treatment plans. The plaintiffs in this case are asserting that these arrangements might discourage people from choosing their own clinical psychologist, contrary to a state statute that provides for freedom of choice.

It is obviously too soon to tell whether these lawsuits will result in the enunciation of liability-expanding doctrines about the incentive and referral arrangement of managed care organizations. What may result from them, however, is an increased emphasis on mechanisms to detect under-utilization of health care where payment and referral arrangements create such incentives.

Refusal to Consent to Psychotropic Drugs

Most states adhere to the same general principles concerning psychiatric patient consent. In brief, those principles are: (1) admission to a psychiatric or substance abuse treatment facility is not an adjudication of mental incompetence, so that psychiatric and substance abuse patients are deemed competent to make treatment decisions unless proven otherwise; (2) if a patient is in fact incompetent, a guardian must be appointed to make treatment decisions, or some other surrogate decision-making arrangements must be made; and (3) surrogate decision-makers use either the "substituted judgment" approach, whereby they seek to arrive at the same decision the patient would make, or the "best interest" approach, which tries to act from an objective viewpoint without reference to the patient's inferred preferences.

These principles are often reflected in laws about patients' rights. They generally provide that, in addition to retaining their rights and privileges as citizens, patients also have the right to participate in their care. About half the states have statutes that give patients the right to refuse medication (Herman, 1989). Some states prescribe what information must be disclosed to the patient about the medications, and require a particular form of consent document.

The two leading court decisions on the issue of the right to refuse psychotropic medications agree that voluntary competent psychiatric patients have an absolute right to refuse such medications, but disagree as to whether active judicial involvement is required to determine the patient's incapacity to make such a decision. The Supreme Court has not addressed the issue squarely, but did hold that the Constitution requires a physician making treatment decisions about an institutionalized retarded person to exercise professional judgment. (This rather lenient "professional judgment" standard has been adopted by some courts in the context of decisions to release voluntary psychiatric patients.) Most states have interpreted the federal court decisions to mean that prior judicial approval for the use of psychotropic drugs on a refusing involuntary patient is not required.

In the managed care setting, this question of a patient's refusal to consent to psychotropic drugs centers on the question of coverage. Involuntary inpatients who refuse medications are subject to the legal doctrines found in the case law summarized above. Voluntary patients who disagree with the treatment plan are free to terminate treatment and/or leave the facility, unless meeting the applicable legal standard for commitment. Voluntary patients who are not committable and who refuse to consent present a problem to managed care entities that can be largely resolved through the inclusion of careful language in the enrollee's contract with the plan.

A subscriber contract, for example, might explicitly acknowledge the patient's right to disagree with clinical decisions. The contract would clearly state that in such a case, the plan has no further obligation to provide the care in question, that the patient is free to seek the care from another provider at his own expense, and that the plan has no obligation for the cost or outcome of such care. The contract should also state that in this type of disagreement, the patient may utilize the plan's member grievance process.

Given the variety of state statues governing the consent to mental health treatment, it is difficult to generalize about what will most effectively protect the managed care entity from liability. It appears however, that the type of contract provision indicated above, together with careful adherence to the various state-mandated procedures governing commitment, adjudication of incompetence (or inability to make treatment decisions), guardianship and informed consent, will help.

Protection From Harm

The potential liability for failing to protect mental health patients or their victims from harm has increased for several reasons. The standard for involuntary commitment has been raised, making it more difficult to commit a potentially dangerous patient. Many states now require that patients be treated in the least restrictive setting possible. State laws increasingly emphasize the rights of psychiatric patients. In light of these developments, managed mental health organizations are understandably concerned about potential expansions of the duty to protect patients and others based on the *Tarasoff* decision. Combined with the legal theories relied upon by the plaintiffs in the *Wilson* case, it could impose duties on persons indirectly involved in treatment decisions.

The landmark decision of *Tarasoff* vs. *Regents of the University of California* established a psychotherapist's duty to use reasonable care to protect a patient's intended victim if the therapist determines that the patient presents a serious danger to an *identified* potential victim. A California appellate court has carefully distinguished the *Tarasoff* creation of an affirmative duty owed to an identified person from a statutory exception to the psychotherapist-patient privilege that does not require a readily identifiable victim. Nevertheless, some courts have expanded the *Tarasoff* duty to protect to situations where certain persons would likely be victims if the patient became violent. In the case of *Hamman* vs. *County of Maricopa,* for example, the Arizona Supreme Court adopted a "zone of danger" test, so that the psychiatrist has a duty to exercise reasonable care to protect the persons within that zone who are the foreseeable victims of the patient. At least one court has imposed liability where the danger is to the public at large rather than any particular person. In Kentucky, a statute has been enacted imposing a duty on a therapist to warn known endangered persons. On the other hand, some states do not impose a duty to protect even where a potential victim has been identified.

While state courts and legislatures debate the question of whether there is a duty to protect and to whom the duty is owed, the managed mental health entity is also concerned with who owes the duty. One such issue has to do with health professionals such as professional counselors and social workers, who are part of the treatment team and who may be in a position to assess the patient's propensity to violence. As cost containment pressures increase, so too will the impetus to use these lower-cost professionals for relatively less acute patients.

If the duty to protect is extended to include all mental health professionals who are employed by an HMO or other managed care entity, it may give rise to the entity's vicarious liability under the respondeat superior theory. It does not take very much imagination to also foresee the potential for the direct corporate liability of a mental health plan for failure to institute adequate policies and procedures designed to carry out the duty to protect, once the potential danger posed by a plan member becomes know to the plan.

Who owes a duty to protect third parties from mental health patients can depend on where and how those patients are treated. Many courts have reasoned that the duty to protect depends upon the existence of a "special relationship" between the defendant and patient. The special relationship incorporates the ability to restrain or control the patient's behavior. If the patient is receiving care at a non-residential outpatient treatment center (e.g., an alcohol rehabilitation center), no liability for the patient's behavior would likely arise since neither the center nor its personnel would have the degree of custodial control over the patient that is a hallmark of the special relationship required for the existence of a duty to protect.

These potential liabilities place a premium on good communications among all those in the managed mental health delivery system (Fortin, 1989). Everyone on the treatment team should inform the PCP or primary therapist of any indication that a patient is dangerous. Once the danger has been established, the potential victims, and perhaps local law enforcement officials, should be contacted. If the patient has seen several mental health practitioners, it is vital that a complete and continuous medical record be maintained so that the current treatment team is aware of all relevant facts. If an outpatient treatment plan includes the use of medication to control the patient's propensity for violence, adherence to that plan should be carefully monitored.

Another area of potential liability centers on the protection of the mental health patient from the employees of the health care provider and from fellow patients. Courts have commonly ruled that the standards of care imposed on the mental health provider differ with the degree of control the employer exercises over its employees and other patients. In a recent Indiana case (*Stopes* vs. *The Heritage House Children's Center of Shelbyville, Inc.*), however, an extraordinary standard of care was imposed on an inpatient mental health facility which made the facility liable for the acts of its employees regardless of whether those acts fell within the scope of their employment. This extended duty was imposed because the facility undertook to control the environment of a patient who was entirely dependent on the facility, a situation analogous to the duty owed by common carriers, such as airlines, to their passengers.

CONCLUSION

It is clear that the advent of managed mental health raises a number of important legal issues. Some of these have been adjudicated in the general health care arena but the extent to which they affect mental health is not yet clear. Others, specific to managed mental health will be identified and adjudicated as the field continues to grow. Still others, such as anti-trust, are common to all business entities. Whatever their source or degree of specialty, managed mental health entities will inevitably be confronted by a number of legal issues that will have a significant effect on the pace and nature of their development.

REFERENCES

BCBSA Survey, Prepared by the Office of Governmental Relations, State Services Departments, Blue Cross and Blue Shield Association, 1989.

Blum, J.: An analysis of legal liability in health care utilization review and case management. *Houston L. Rev., 18:*199–200, 1989.

Case abstract of Noto v. St. Vincent's Hospital, *Medical Liability Reporter, 11:*64, 1989.

Fox, P.: Foreword: Overview of managed care trends. In: *The Insider's Guide to Managed Care; A Legal and Operational Roadmap,* 1:3. National Health Lawyers Association, 1990.

Fortin, J.: Legal trends and issues for mental health providers. In (A. Gosfield, ed.), *Health Law Handbook.* New York, Clark Boardman, 1989.

Herman, D.: The basis for the right of committed patients to refuse psychotropic medication. *J. Health and Hospital Law, 22:*176–177, 1989.

Kenkel, P.: More physicians joining IPAs to compete with specialty groups over managed care. *Modern Healthcare, 19:*32, 1989.

Kunnes, R.: Viewpoints: Managed psych care, quality under experts' microscopes. *Managed Care Outlook, 2:*7, 1989.

Mullen, P.: PPO's: Will the boom continue? *Managed HealthCare,* 10–11, 1989.

Mullen, P.: Oregon psychologists sue HMO. *Managed HealthCare, 1:*9, 1989.

Rolph, E., Rich, J.P., Ginsburg, P., Hosek, S., Keenan, K., and Gertler, G.: *State Laws and Regulations Governing Preferred Provider Organizations,* 8–11, Rand Corporation, 1986.

AUTHOR INDEX

Patrick, D., 66, 80
Paul, M., 241
Pearson, J., viii, xviii, xxiii, 127
Peebles, T., 242
Pelletier, L., 243
Penzer, W., 118, 124
Pereira, J., 106, 124
Petrocine, W., 221
Piersma, H., 243
Pion, K., 43
Pope, C., 242
Price, K., 241
Price, S., 213, 221
Prospero, A., 121, 124
Prosser, P., 104, 124
Pulice, R., 58

R

Raelin, J., 10, 26
Raphael, B., 237, 243
Reed, S., 49, 57
Reich, P., 231, 243
Reich, W., 245, 257, 263
Reinhardt, U., 248, 256, 265
Relman, A., 21, 26, 248, 257, 263, 264, 265
Rich, J., viii, xviii, xxiii, 267, 290
Rinaldo, D., 142
Rivlin, L., 240, 243
Roberts, R., 73, 81
Robins, L., 225, 243
Rodin, B., 116, 124
Rogers, W., 73, 82
Rolph, E., 271, 290
Rosenthanl, E., 251, 255, 257, 263
Rosie, J., 243
Rothbard, A., viii, xxiii, 45, 48, 49, 52, 54, 55, 56, 58, 59
Russell, G., 238, 243
Rutter, M., 239, 243
Ryan, P., 215, 221

S

Sabin, J., 265
Santiago, J., 236, 243
Sarnat, J., 213, 221
Saxe, L., 230, 234, 243
Schene, A., 233, 243

Schinnar, A., viii, xxiii, 45, 48, 52, 54, 55, 56, 58, 59
Schlesinger, M., 55, 56, 59, 70, 81
Schroeder, S., 221
Schuckit, M., 234, 243
Schwartz, I., 240
Schwel, M., 243
Seigler, M., 264
Seltzer, D., 74, 81
Shadle, M., 43, 105, 124, 228, 243
Shapiro, R., 97
Sharfstein, S., 46, 59, 76, 81
Shelp, E., 265
Shemo, J., 225, 244
Sherbourne, C., 73, 82
Shore, M., 48, 57
Shumwag, M., 98
Siddall, L., 73, 81
Sjodin, I., 235, 244
Smith, J., 117, 124
Smith, J.C.H., ix, xviii, xxiii, 165, 169, 181, 192, 199
Smith, J.R., 221
Smith, H., 178, 199
Smith, N., 207, 221
Smith, M., 233, 234
Snyder, T. Jr., 220
Solloway, J., 69, 74, 80
Solovitz, B., 54, 58
Somers, S., 48, 57
Soreff, S., 244
Spencer, J., 238, 244
Spitzer, R., 98
Spoerl, O., 66, 81
Stanley, J., 178, 199
Starr, P., 62, 63, 64, 71, 81, 248, 257, 265
Staver, S., 248, 250, 265
Stein, L., 90, 98
Stein, R., 244
Stoeckle, J., 255, 264
Subramanian, K., 244
Surles, R., 50, 53, 57, 59
Svedlund, J., 235, 244

T

Talbott, J., 46, 56, 59, 90
Tarini, P., 118, 124
Taub, H., 235, 241

SUBJECT INDEX

A

Absenteeism, 106, 118, 189
Access
    to data, 145, 150, 151, 153, 154, 155, 157, 159, 160, 161
    to services, 6, 13, 23, 28, 35, 41, 50, 55, 65, 66, 69, 115, 131, 134, 135, 136, 138, 139, 165, 173, 174, 175, 177, 187, 224, 226, 227, 228, 240, 247, 248, 257, 260, 270, 271, 281
Accessibility, 13, 61, 79, 109, 154, 268
Accountability, xii, 13, 14, 26, 52, 209, 255, 257, 262
Acute care, 21, 46, 55, 210
Adolescents, xix, 119, 122, 133, 185, 192, 213, 227, 240, 242, 243
    admission to inpatient facilities, 31, 32, 83, 102, 128, 176, 226, 228, 239
Affordability, 65, 76, 79
Aftercare, 15, 17, 50, 77, 118, 132, 133, 141, 216
Antitrust, xix, 267, 274, 276, 277, 279, 289
Appeals, 9, 138, 141, 169, 254, 280, 282
Autonomy (*see also* Ethics), 5, 6, 13, 23, 41, 71, 72, 205, 246, 250, 252, 253, 254, 255, 256, 257, 258, 259, 260, 261, 262, 264

B

Benefit(s), xi, 4, 13, 17, 18, 25, 28, 33, 37, 39, 41, 42, 65, 66, 68, 69, 81, 83, 112, 118, 122, 124, 130, 131–133, 134, 138, 153, 163, 167, 172, 214, 224, 244, 245, 247, 256, 258, 259, 262, 273, 274, 280, 282, 283, 284, 285
    design, 98, 106, 111, 114, 119, 120, 136–137
    cuts, 19, 20, 28
    limits, 72, 73, 74, 79, 84, 103, 105, 115, 168, 171, 225, 226, 231
    mandated, 45, 74, 94, 102, 113–114, 123, 128, 215, 223, 226, 268, 270, 287
    protection, xv, 11, 12, 22
    retirees, 30
    substitution, 11, 12, 15, 51, 53, 55, 56, 57, 65, 111, 112, 189, 190
Biological psychiatry, xiii
Biopsychosocial, 223

C

Capitation, 36, 38, 46–59, 76, 77, 229, 253, 272, 274, 277, 278, 285
Case management, xiii, 10, 14, 23, 29, 32, 35, 38, 49, 50, 51, 53, 54, 55, 56, 58, 59, 84, 88, 90, 91, 92, 106, 107, 108, 109, 110, 111, 112, 113, 117, 118, 119, 123, 125, 132, 133, 143, 150, 152, 155, 160, 161, 166, 168, 170, 189, 193, 215, 216, 217, 219, 247, 249, 260, 262, 268, 282, 290
Catchment area, 45, 225
Certificate of need, xi, 247
CHAMPUS, xviii, 94, 175, 192, 211
Channeling, 143
Children, xix, 47, 73, 80, 83, 110, 128, 133, 169, 172, 239, 241, 242, 243, 244, 289
Chronic mentally ill, 46, 47, 48, 49, 50, 51, 56, 58, 59
Claims, 7, 40, 83, 107, 109, 110, 112, 113, 114, 120, 136, 137, 139, 140, 141, 143, 147, 148, 150, 152, 153, 155, 163, 169, 170, 171, 180, 181, 198, 199, 211, 229, 245, 256, 257, 283
Coding, 145, 150, 154, 158
Coinsurance, 28, 34, 37, 84, 105, 113, 134, 137, 271
Community mental health, xviii, 12, 16, 55, 59, 80, 213, 221, 223, 243
    centers, 45, 66, 68, 108

Quality (*continued*)
  external, 216–217
  safeguards, 8–12

R

Rationing, 76, 78, 81, 123
Readmission, 53, 141, 191
Recidivism, 17, 114, 117, 118, 120, 176
Records, 9, 143, 145, 146, 150, 151, 153, 155, 157, 158, 165, 169, 174, 175, 260, 270, 271, 278
Regulatory (*see also* Legal), xviii, 20, 21, 51, 64, 84, 95, 96, 97, 102, 135, 215, 216, 221, 248, 265, 267, 268, 269, 271, 272, 273
Relapse, 117, 129, 236
Relative value scale, 32, 128, 157, 171, 172, 194, 203, 209, 213, 249
Replicability, 167
Research, xvii, 6, 8, 16, 18, 19, 20, 22, 25, 35, 43, 57, 58, 74, 83, 85–87, 89–91, 94, 98, 99, 104, 178, 190, 199, 211–213, 223, 225, 228–231, 233, 235–237, 239, 242, 258
Residential care, 46, 90, 169, 173, 194
Rights, 63, 91, 95, 96, 97, 279, 282, 286, 287
Risk, 17, 28, 36, 38, 40, 42, 46, 49, 50, 51, 52, 53, 54, 55, 56, 66, 68, 69, 71, 77, 88, 90, 114, 116, 119, 138, 143, 179, 193, 205, 206, 207, 208, 210, 213, 215, 216, 217, 218, 220, 221, 223, 228, 230, 231, 232, 237, 243, 253, 269, 272, 273, 274, 275, 276, 277, 278, 279, 281, 284, 285

S

Screening, 34, 49, 143, 169, 170, 171, 175, 202, 206, 208, 215, 216, 217, 218
Second opinion, 32, 145, 149, 150, 153, 155, 160, 161
Self-insured, 11, 17
Social workers, 14, 74, 109, 110, 132, 170, 225, 270, 288
Specialty review, 35
Staff, 13, 15, 16, 19, 24, 65, 66, 104, 106, 110, 115, 116, 131, 133, 136, 137, 139, 143, 144, 145, 146, 147, 148, 149, 151, 152, 153, 154, 155, 156, 157, 158, 159, 160, 162, 166, 169, 171, 175, 205, 206, 207, 208, 209, 210, 221, 277, 280

Staff model, 9, 10, 36, 38, 39, 64, 69, 77
  effect on inpatient utilization, 24
Standards (*see also* Criteria, Protocols), 5, 9, 10, 14, 38, 71, 91, 93–97, 109, 111, 118, 120, 143, 201–205, 207, 208, 211, 212, 215–220, 247, 248, 256, 259, 267, 268, 273, 278, 283, 284, 289
State psychiatric hospitals, 45, 50
Stigma, xiii, 101, 234
Structured outpatient, 15, 17, 107, 157
Substance abuse, xi, 3, 4, 5, 11, 12, 13, 15, 16, 17, 18, 22, 23, 28, 29, 35, 37, 38, 40, 41, 42, 73, 74, 81, 83, 101, 102, 103, 104, 105, 106, 107, 108, 109, 110, 112, 113, 114, 115, 116, 118, 119, 120, 121, 122, 123, 127, 128, 129, 130, 131, 132, 133, 134, 135, 136, 137, 141, 169, 223, 224, 225, 226, 228, 230, 231, 233, 234, 235, 239, 240, 241, 267, 269, 270, 272, 274, 285, 286
Suicide, 193, 210, 221, 231, 232, 241, 243, 244, 283, 284
Supply side, xiii, 84, 85, 87

T

Third party administrator (TPA), 271
Training, xix, 16, 66, 68, 75, 106, 146, 160, 167, 169, 270
Treatment planning, xix, 14, 23, 35, 76, 155, 214, 215
Triage, 93, 109, 110, 116, 117, 118

U

Underpricing, 71
Undertreatment, 71, 88
Underutilization, 47, 214, 216, 217, 218, 219, 234
Union, 13, 18, 30, 37, 65, 135, 215, 271, 273
Utilization, xiii, 9, 12, 16, 17, 19, 24, 39, 49, 50, 53, 58, 69, 73, 74, 80, 81, 83, 84, 86, 87, 88, 90, 91, 92, 94, 97, 101–104, 107–110, 112, 113, 114, 115, 116, 119, 120, 127, 130, 140, 142, 160, 162, 171, 173–174, 184, 185, 187, 193, 198, 199, 221, 224, 225, 226, 227, 229, 230, 232, 234, 235, 241, 242, 243, 247, 248, 255, 256, 257, 264, 267, 271, 278
Utilization control (*see* Utilization review)

Utilization management (*see* Utilization
  review)
Utilization review, 19, 21, 26, 29, 34, 36, 40,
  42, 43, 68, 83, 97, 98, 105, 106, 109, 118,
  122, 123, 124, 128, 129, 132, 133, 139, 141,
  143, 144–149, 153–158, 163, 166, 169, 170,
  172, 175, 181, 186, 203, 208, 213, 214, 215,
  219, 253, 272, 276, 277, 281, 283, 284, 290
  concurrent, 7, 32, 35, 84, 88, 89, 91, 94, 198,
    209, 210, 221, 254, 282, 285

retrospective, 7, 32, 68, 107, 110, 162, 205,
  206, 209, 210, 253, 282

V

Value, 5, 7, 13, 21, 30, 32, 72, 78, 79, 95, 147,
  167, 180, 186, 201, 206, 235, 238, 242, 245,
  246, 258
Values, 9, 10, 66, 72, 202, 246, 251
Variance, 168, 184, 204, 282